ANAL AND PERIANAL LESIONS

**PROF. P. SIVALINGAM
DR. S. VADAMALAYAN**

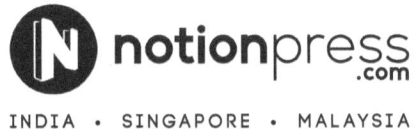

INDIA • SINGAPORE • MALAYSIA

Notion Press

No. 8, 3rd Cross Street
CIT Colony, Mylapore
Chennai, Tamil Nadu – 600004

First Published by Notion Press 2021
Copyright © Prof. P. Sivalingam & Dr. S. Vadamalayan 2021
All Rights Reserved.

ISBN 978-1-63832-759-2

This book has been published with all efforts taken to make the material error-free after the consent of the author. However, the author and the publisher do not assume and hereby disclaim any liability to any party for any loss, damage, or disruption caused by errors or omissions, whether such errors or omissions result from negligence, accident, or any other cause.

While every effort has been made to avoid any mistake or omission, this publication is being sold on the condition and understanding that neither the author nor the publishers or printers would be liable in any manner to any person by reason of any mistake or omission in this publication or for any action taken or omitted to be taken or advice rendered or accepted on the basis of this work. For any defect in printing or binding the publishers will be liable only to replace the defective copy by another copy of this work then available.

CONTENTS

Unique Feature of The Book	5
About the Authors	7
Forwarded	11
Preface	15
CHAPTER 1: Setting up Colo Rectal Clinic and Examination of Ano Rectal Lesions	17
CHAPTER 2: Ano Rectal Trauma	29
CHAPTER 3: Functional Anorectal Pain	37
CHAPTER 4: Fissure in Ano	43
CHAPTER 5: Haemorrhoids	59
CHAPTER 6: Anorectal Suppuration	87
CHAPTER 7: Fistula in Ano	99
CHAPTER 8: Pruritus Ani	121
CHEPTER 9: Complications of Anal Surgery	129
CHAPTER 10: Anal Stenosis	137
CHAPTER 11: Faecal Incontinence	147

CHAPTER 12: Bacterial Synergisic Infection — 163

CHAPTER 13: Perianal Hidradinitis Suppuration (PHS) — 171

CHAPTER 14: Anal Condylomata — 179

CHAPTER 15: Anorectal Lesions in HIV Patients — 187

CHAPTER 16: Anal Intraepithelial Neoplasia (AIN) — 197

CHAPTER 17: Carcinoma of Anal Region — 205

UNIQUE FEATURE OF THE BOOK

The author of this book had training in Colo-Rectal Surgery in LEEDS GENERAL INFIRMARY –Leeds and in St MARKS HOSPITAL London for one year under Common Wealth Medical Fellowship. After return from training, he started the Colorectal department in Govt. Rajaji Hospital Madurai. The final year M.B;B.S; students, Internees, and Post Graduates in General Surgery were posted in Colorectal out patients clinic. With periodical interaction with the students, many of them of are of opinion that a book exclusively for the lesions in the anal and Perianal region with basic aspect of preoperative preparation for the colorectal surgery will be more helpful for them. Keeping in mind from the feedback by the trainee from different categories, the topic were selected. The chapters are carefully selected to complete the lesions in the anal and Perianal region as per the demand by the trainees. So this book has come on demand to fulfilment of the surgical trainees.

ABOUT THE AUTHORS

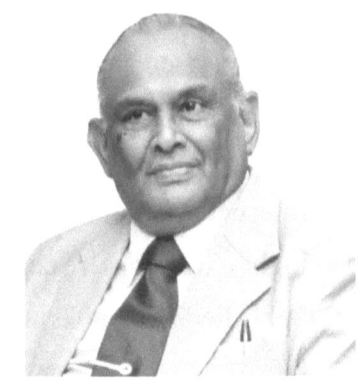

Professor P. Sivalingam. M.S; M.N.A.M.S

1. Retd. Professor and Head of the Department of Surgery, Madurai Medical College and Colorectal Surgeon Govt. Rajaji Hospital Madurai.
2. Common Wealth Medical Fellowship Award in Colo Rectal Surgery in 1981- 1982.
3. Governing Council Member of The Tamil Nadu Dr. M.G.R. Medical University for 3 years from August 2000.
4. President of Association of Colon and Rectal Surgeons of India for two years (1995-1996).
5. Chairman Tamil Nadu and Pondicherry chapter of Association of Surgeons of India in 1998.
6. Director of Surgical Studies in Association of Surgeons of India for 3 years (2001 – 2003)

7. Chairman Board of Examination for Fellowship of Association of Colon and Rectal Surgeons of India (2008 – 2011)
8. President of Ostomates India, Madurai Chapter (1994 – 2015)
9. Fellow of International Society of Coloproctology (2014).
10. Lectures were given in 92 topics in various places in India.
11. Faculty in 35 Seminars and 10 Workshops.
12. Lectures were given in 47 Continuous Medical Programs.
13. Member in 13 academic bodies in medical field.
14. A total of 29 Scientific papers were published in National and International Journals.
15. Eight chapters were contributed in different medical books.
16. Published five books so far.
17. Life time Achievement Award received from:
    i. Asian Federation of Coloproctology (2009)
    ii. Association of Colon and Rectal Surgeons of India (2009)
    iii. The Tamil Nadu Dr. M.G.R. Medical University (2012)
18. Examiner for Surgery in various Universities in southern States of India and National Board of Examinations

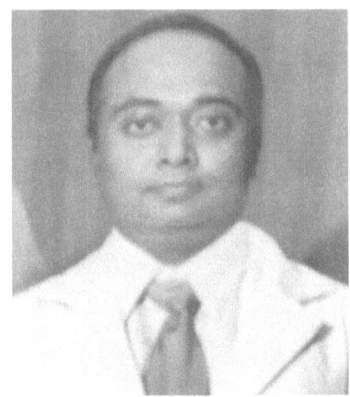

Dr. Vadamalayan .S
MD FACS
Drvadu@yahoo.com

1. Internship in General Surgery North shore Long Island Jewish Hospital
2. General Surgery Residency New York Methodist Hospital
3. Highest Academic Award New York methodist hospital 2007
4. American Board of Surgery certification 2013
5. Fellow of American College of Surgeons 2020
6. Surgeon at Interfaith Medical Center New York
7. Membership is American College of Surgeons ,American medical association and Medical Society of New York
8. Factors affecting patient disposition after laparoscopic adjustable gastric banding (LAGB): Analysis of bariatric outcome longitudinal database .97th Annual American college of surgeons 2011.
9. Fate of retained capule: pathogonomic for surgery". Am. Surg 2007
10. Contributed to four chapters in Topics in Colo Rectal Surgery Book

FORWARDED

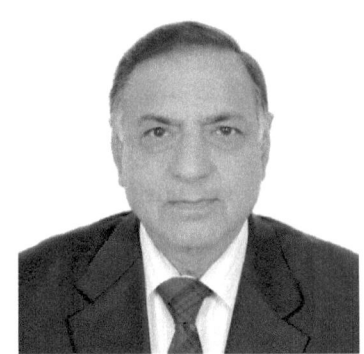

DR. VIJAY ARORA, MS., FRCS., FACRS.
INTERNATIONAL ADVICER. RCPSG
CHAIRMAN DEPARTMENT OF SURGERY AND LAPAROSCOPIC SURGERY
SURGEON IN CHARGE OF COLORECTAL UNIT
SIR GANGA RAM HOSPITAL, NEW DELHI

Dr. P. Sivalingam ponniah is a veteran colo-proctologist surgeon with decades of experience. It is my privilege and honour to write a foreword for his book "Anal and Perianal lesions".

The book is written in his inimical style with reflection of a lifetime of experience in the process of training and practicing the art of colo-rectal surgery. He brings his depth of knowledge and wisdom gained through a lifetime. The book addresses all surgeons who wish to pursue the surgery of anal and perianal lesions from the basics to the most recent advances along with practical tips and suggestions. The explanations bring out the finer details of day to day practice in a very simplified format.

I found the book to be a wealth of guidance and it is a handbook to consult when any ticklish situation arises and is encountered by younger colleagues.

Dr. P. Sivalingam has poured his knowledge and distilled his wisdom with a lifetime of experience to bring a roadmap through explanatory details and illustrated diagrams. This will be of use to all pursing colorectal surgery. I commend this book to all aspiring to attain a proficiency in the practice of colo-rectal surgery as a valuable adjunct and guide.

Dr. Vijay Arora

Date: 10.01.2021

Place: New Delhi

Dr. Shantikumar Chivate

M.S., F.C.P.S., F.I.C.S., F.A.C.R.S.I., F.I.S.C.P.

Surgeon (R No. 25458)

Forwarded :

Dr. P. Sivalingam is to be congratulated on his successful completion of the second book of Colon and Rectal Surgery. The contents have been changed to reflect recent changes in the Core factors in treatment of colorectal surgery. Clinical material is useful for young surgeons training residents in colon and rectal surgery and new practicing surgeons starting their carrier find themselves stranded and are in need of a comprehensive guide which provides all essential components of colorectal surgery. At least one third of the material has been completely renewed to reflect advances in the science of colorectal surgery. The book will rapidly become a major resource for training, read by almost all trainees, budding surgeons interested in colo rectal specialty. The purpose of the book was originally to provide a standardized reference for evidence-based recommendations. The book a success and should be considered a major selfless contribution to our society and specialty by Dr. P. Sivalingam. As time passes, our specialty and its knowledge surrounding it certainly change, existence of this book and the details which perpetuates it guarantees that we always have the most up-to-date information. The Executive Council of the International Society of Coloproctology is fully supportive of this effort by Dr. Sivalingam and gratefully recognizes his contribution. Please remember the sacrifice of time and effort that made this publication possible. Strive to add to the knowledge which one day changes our practice and our specialty on colorectal disease as we improve patient care.

President : International Society of Coloproctology

Special Interest : General Surgery, Laser-Piles, Fistula, Colorectal Surgery, Cancer Surgery, Varicose Vein Laser Tre Diabetic Foot & Non Healing Wound, Prolapse Rectum, Severe Constipation, Elephantiasis

Tel. : 022-2538 0778, 2540 6465, Mobile : 9869168730
Jeevan Jyot Hospital, Satyam Apartments, Opp. Shahu Market, Near Naupada Police Station, Naupada, Thane (W) 4
E-mail : shantikumar@drchivate.com / drshantikumar@gmail.com

www.drchivat

PREFACE

'People who change after change will survive. People who change with the change will succeed. People who cause change will lead'.

Doctors who got training in colorectal surgery abroad and in India in nineteen eighties felt the need for specialization in colorectal surgery in India. For this purpose, The Association of Colon and Rectal Surgeons of India, and the International Society of Colo Proctology, are conducting C.M.E. Workshop, and hand on training every year in India in different places. The Colorectal surgery is now advancing in all respect and sub specialization may develop in future shortly. Keeping in mind about the vast development in colorectal surgery this book on Lesions of Anal and Perianal Region is focussing on common conditions in the Anal and Perianal Region, stressing on the basic aspects of the diseases and recent advances in pathogenesis and management.

The topic on setting up of colorectal clinic is mainly for those who want to start colorectal clinic exclusively, as a guideline, though it will not come in the heading of this book. Bacterial synergistic infection in the Perianal region may spread as a life threatening condition is discussed in an elaborate way to save the life and to reduce the complications. Most of the patients attending the colorectal clinic have disturbances in defecation either constipation or incontinence. Constipation, in most of the cases can be managed by nonsurgical way, incontinence may need surgical managed. So incontinence is discussed. With modern treatment,

HIV infected persons are living for longer time and Anorectal lesions in HIV patients are common and so they are discussed as a separate topic.

This book, I am sure, will be a review for the surgical practioners, postgraduate trainees, and teachers, about the pathophysiology, diagnosis and management of the lesions of anal and Perianal region and will offer a complete range of therapeutic options. It is up to the reader to get the best of everything in this book. This book aims to provide the benefits and outcome of one of the most rewarding but potentially dangerous area of surgical practice where the surgeons name and fame may be damaged. Despite of advanced medical technology, skilful hands and brilliant mind, we have our human limitations.

In a way, criticism actually helps one to walk on the path of perfection. Therefore, feedback both positive and negative are appreciated.

Dr. P. Sivalingam. M.S; M.N.A.M.S

Email: drpsivalingam@yahoo.com

Cell: 88700 55855

Date: 16.03.2021

CHAPTER 1

SETTING UP COLO RECTAL CLINIC AND EXAMINATION OF ANO RECTAL LESIONS

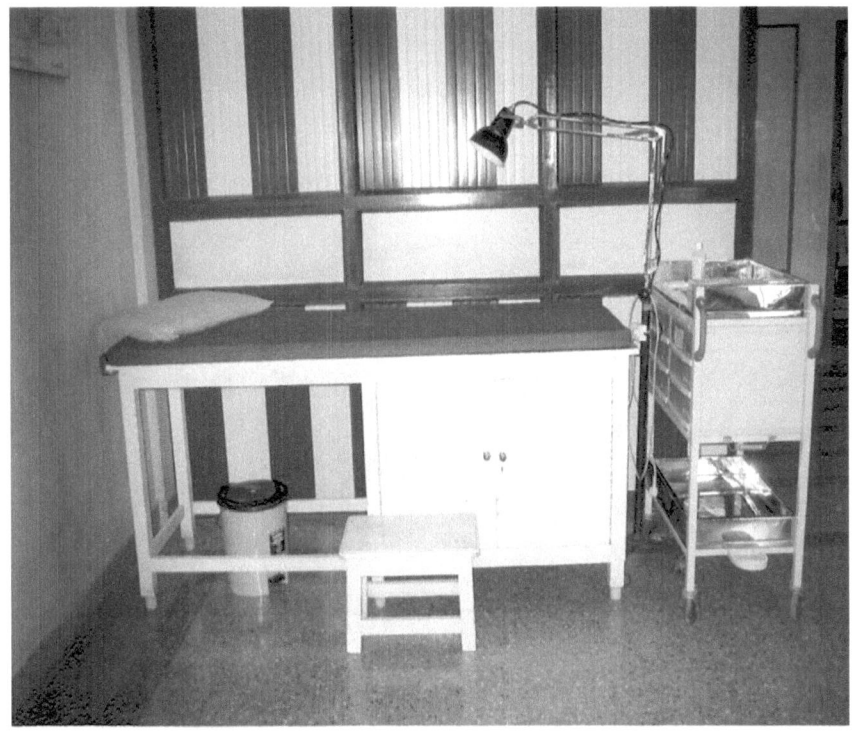

1.01. Examination couch

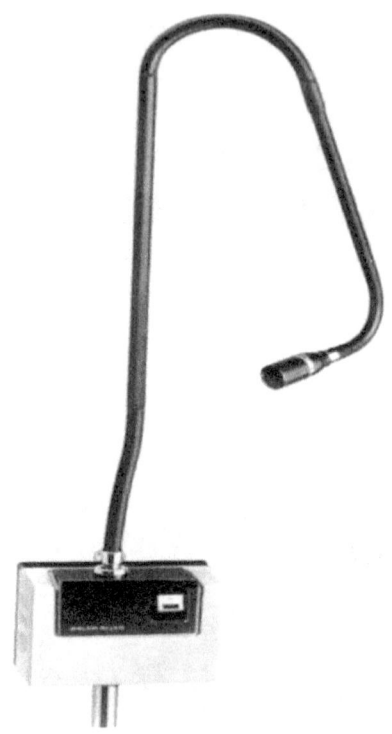

1.02. Halogen lamp with malleable arm

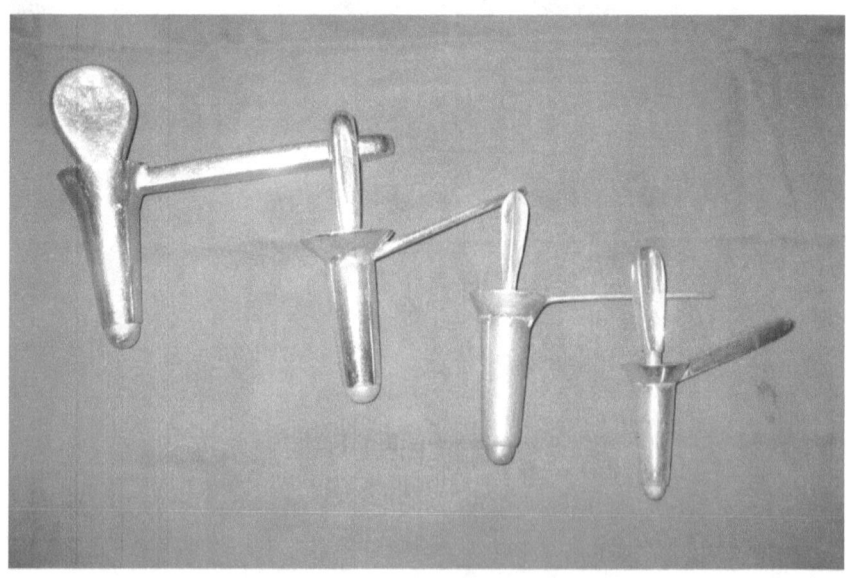

1.03. Different types of proctoscope

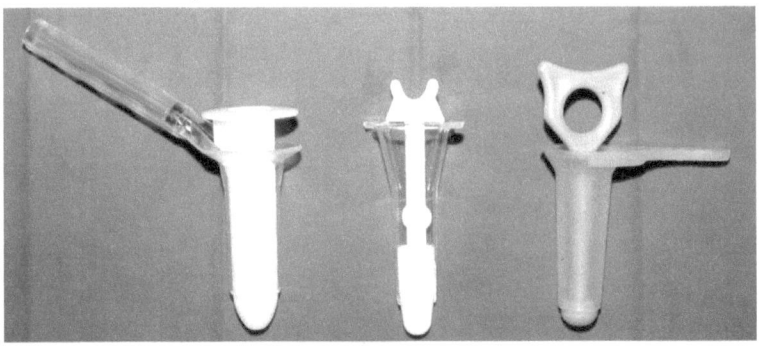

1.04. Disposable proctoscope

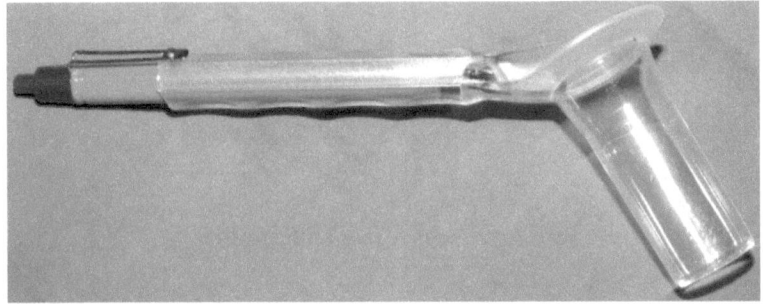

1.05. Self-illuminating proctoscope

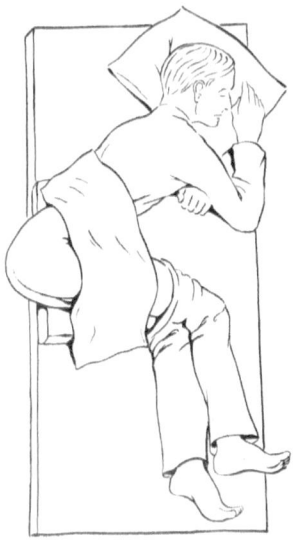

1.06. Left lateral position

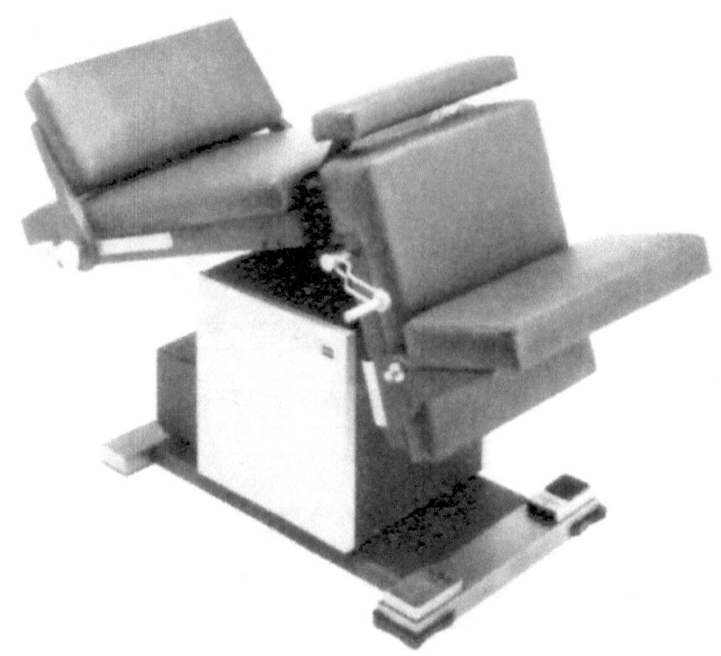

1.07. Ritter table – Jack knife position

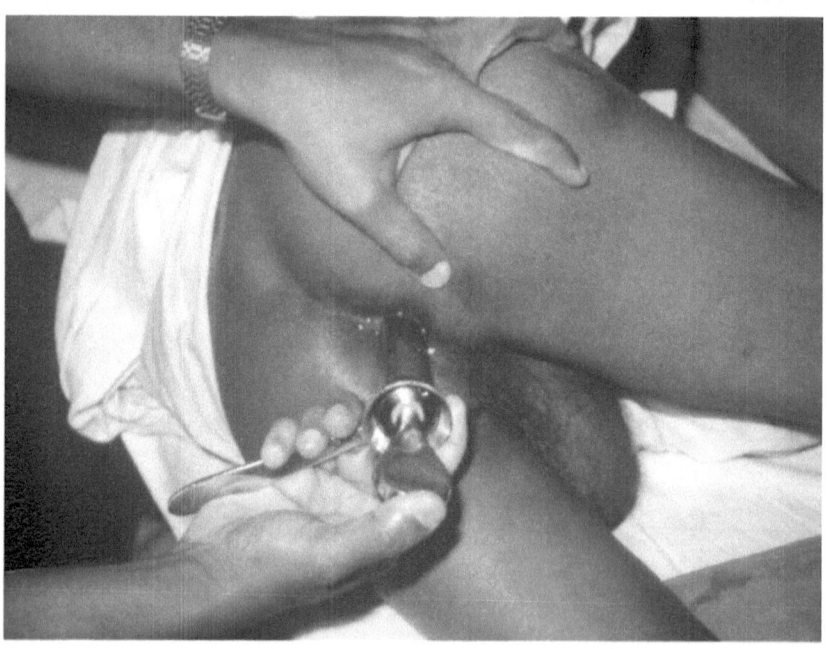

1.08. The way to hold the Proctoscope during proctoscopy

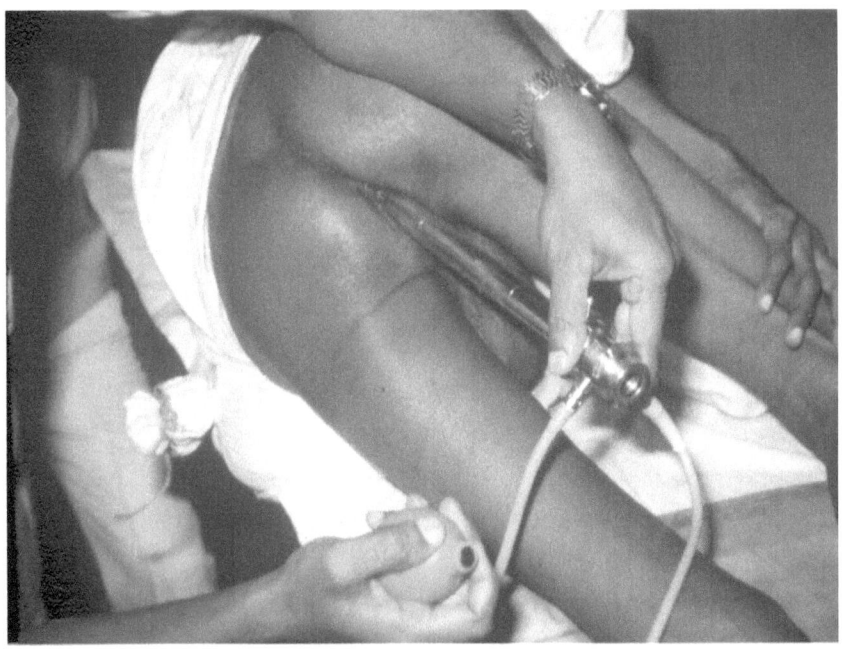

1.09. Sigmoidoscopy- Left hand is resting over patient's right buttock

1. HISTORY OF COLORECTAL SURGERY

Though the surgery of colorectal region has been known and practiced since the down of civilisation, it is only in 19th century the importance of colorectal diseases realised. In 1835, Frederic Salmon established St Marks Hospital in London. Later St Marks Hospital becomes the Mecca for treatment of colon and rectal diseases, was, and continues to be visited by many surgeons throughout the world. Joseph M. Mathew got training in St. Mark's hospital and started colorectal practice in America in 1878.

2. GOOD LIGHT

Good light is essential for the examination of the anal region and the illumination focusing on down to the proctoscope. For this purpose, an angle poise examination lamp is excellent. The bulb should be at least 100 watts. Halogen light can be used for good illumination (fig1.02).

3. GOOD VENTILATION

Good ventilation with exhaust fan provision is essential. The examination room must have a strict privacy for the patient and the examination team.

4. EXAMINATION COUCH

For Ano rectal examination the patient should ideally be on proper examination couch (1.01) the top that must be at least 80 cm from the ground, otherwise, the surgeon will have to stoop unduly. Disposable gloves to be used for rectal examination. Water-soluble lubricant with lignocaine is more convenient for the patient. Petroleum jelly should not be used, as it is difficult to clean from the patient's Perianal skin and to clean the instruments.

5. PROCTOSCOPE

Many different types of proctoscopes are available in length, calibre, and shape (1.03).The larger the sheath of the proctoscope the better will be view obtained. Normally 7 cm long with a diameter of 22 mm in the tip and 32 mm at the base, are commonly used in clinical practice. For patients with painful conditions or with some degree of anal spasm or stenosis a narrow proctoscope should be used. The length of the anal canal varies in patients according the physiques. In some heavy build individuals, the scope cannot be inserted beyond the anal canal. Disposable proctoscope(1.04) self-illuminating proctoscope for diagnosis and treatment are also available (1.05).

6. SIGMOIDOSCOPE

Rigid Sigmoidoscope of different diameters are available. Normally for routine Sigmoidoscopy, 16 mm diameter with 30cm length is used. Long alligator forceps are used for holding swabs to clean out the lumen of the bowel, and biopsy forceps with sharp cupped blades are the integral part for Sigmoidoscpy. Long suction tubes for suction of the liquid faces and profuse discharge as in acute ulcerative colitis is essential when doing sigmoidoscopy.

7. A dressing trolley of 80 x 65 X 45 cm with underneath self-cupboards for keeping all instruments used during the colorectal clinical examination. A number of kidney trays and a bucket for receiving the dirty swabs must be kept in the clinic. Provision must be made to hold the Sigmoidoscope and long alligator forceps which is attached to the trolley in the form of long holder.

8. Equipments for minor surgical procedures like incision and drainage of abscess, biopsy, injection therapy for piles and cauterizing agents like copper sulphate stick and anal dilators for anal stenosis, rubber band ligator etc. must be available in the colorectal clinic for immediate use when required.

9. HISTORY TAKING

The diagnosis of Anorectal diseases depend on a careful assessment of the informations derived from the medical history, rectal examination, proctoscopic, sigmoidoscopic, abdominal and general examination, colonoscopy and other investigations. With some complaints, the diagnosis is virtually evident from the history alone or on very simple physical examination. Rarely even with all latest investigations, it may not be possible to arrive at the conclusion. Under these circumstances, re-examination when the symptoms are maximal or after an interval of sometime may prove helpful.

10. EXAMINATION OF PATIENT WITH ANORECTAL CONDITIONS

In all Anorectal problems, rectal examination is the most important but it is very embaracing experience for the patient. If the patient has pain in the anal region, the patient will be very apprehensive and will have tight anal sphincter and spasm of buttock muscles. If the surgeon proceeds with rectal examination regardless of this, the spasm increases, so the rectal examination becomes extremely difficult. The surgeon's first duty is to allay any anxiety and to encourage the patient to relax his musculature and keep it relaxed throughout the examination. Any attempt to overcome the spasm with undue force, usually hurt the patient and increases the tension of the musculature. An essential feature of gentleness in examinations is the avoidance of instruments that are badly designed. The patient must be warned about the sensation or feeling of passing wind or urgency for stool when rectal examination is being done.

10.1 POSITION OF THE PATIENT

10.1.1. Left lateral position
The left lateral position is the simplest and more satisfactory for all Anorectal conditions (1.06). Patient's buttocks must project a little beyond the edge of the couch. A small sand bag may be placed under the buttocks. The trunk must lie obliquely across the couch top so that the head lies near the opposite edge. The position of the trunk is arranged in such a way that the hips are flexed to about 100 degree and the legs parallel and close is the opposite edge of the couch. The right shoulder is placed a little downward direction, so that there will be a prone inclination for the trunk of the body and this inclination of the body is maintained though out the examination.

10.1.2. Knee Chest position
This position is award and undignified for the patient. The patient may be susceptible to syncope after the examination in this position.

10.1.3. Inverted or Jack Knife position -Ritter table (1.07)
This position is popular in United State and is extremely efficient position for sigmoidoscopy.

11. INSPECTION

This is one of the most neglected parts of the examination of the Anorectal conditions. Lesions like anal fissure, perianal hematoma, and anal warts or pruritus can be diagnosed on inspection alone. When the left hand lift the upper buttock to expose the anus and perianal region, to have a clear view of the Pathological condition like prolapsed piles skin tag, external opening of the fistula, perianal suppuration and lower edge of the carcinoma. In suspected rectal prolapse, it may be necessary to examine the patient during straining on a toilet.

12. RECTAL EXAMINATION

To achieve a satisfactory and reasonably comfortable examination it is essential to inform the patient about what is going to be done. Rectal examination may be unsuccessful if proper explanation is not provided.

12.1. TECHNIQE OF RECTAL EXAMINATION

The gloved index finger is lubricated with water-soluble lubricant and the pulp of the right index finger should be placed gently over the anal orifice and pressure is exerted until the sphincter relaxes allowing the finger to enter. Surrounding structures should be examined in an orderly manner. By rectal examination not only the interior of the rectum and anal canal is palpated, but also the wall and the structures outside the wall are also palpated. Normally the finger will reach up to 7 cm from anal margin. By bushing the perineum, an extra 2-3cm can be reached.

After reaching the upper palpable limit, the finger is withdrawn slowly and feels the whole circumference of the wall of rectum and anal canal and the anterior, posterior, and lateral walls to find out any pathology in the wall or close to the wall outside.

12.2. Anorectal ring:

The Anorectal ring is situated at the junction of the surgical anal canal and the rectum, is a composite fibro muscular band composed of the upper part of the internal sphincter muscle, the longitudinal muscle of the rectum, the puborectalis muscle and the deeper part of external sphincter muscle. The tip of the finger is in level with it when the proximal inter phalange joint is at the anal verge. When the finger is inserted a little further, the distal inter phalangeal joint can be flexed over the upper surface of the Anorectal ring. Running forward from coccyx on either side is the sacrospinous ligament. In men, the prostate and seminal vesicles should be palpated for abnormal firmness, hypertrophy or nodularity. The internal haemorrhoids are normally not palpable but very long standing haemorrhoids associated with fibrosis may be felt as longitudinal ridges of folds. Indurations following injection treatment may remain palpable for several weeks. Bidigital examination of the ano rectal region and perianal structures is essential to find out the course of fistula tract.

When a tumour is palpated, its position, size and whether it is ulcerated, sessile or, polyphoidal in nature and the depth of the bowel wall involvement, mobility, fixity, and its involvement in relation to the circumference of the bowel and the distance from anal margin are carefully noted and documented.

12.3. In female the Cervix of the uterus should not be mistaken for a tumour which is more commonly occurs when the cervix is irregular.

13. PROCTOSCOPY

No special bowel preparation is required for proctoscope.

Select the size of the proctospe for the individual case, depending upon the digital examination findings. The proctoscope is smeared with water-soluble lubricant (1.08). It is held in right hand with the thumb over the obturator handle and gently introduced to the anal canal and gently pushed in the direction of umbilicus until the proctoscope tip enters the lower 3rd of the rectum. This is appreciated by diminished resistance to the passage of the proctoscope.

14. SIGMOIDOSCOPY

Rigid Sigmoidoscope of different diameters and lengths are available. Normally 16mm diameter and 30 cm length scope is used. Pre examination enema is usually not necessary and pre examination enema actually has some drawbacks.

a. The content of the enema may be irritant to the rectal mucosa and may cause mucus discharge which may give raise to confusion in diagnosis.

b. If there is no complete return of enema fluid, the rectum and Sigmoid colon will be loaded with liquid faeces. The liquid faeces are much more difficult for Sigmoidoscopic examination than loaded solid or semi-solid faces. In other words, inefficient preparation is much worse than no preparation at all.

14.1. TECHNIQUE OF SIGMOIDOSCOPY

Normally no anaesthesia is required for sigmoidoscopy. Patient in left lateral position, the surgeons left forearm should rest on the patient's right buttock (1.09) to have control over the movements of the instrument and to safeguard in case when the scope moves suddenly. Well-lubricated scope is introduced through the anus and first directed towards the umbilicus and later towards the sacrum. The lower rectum and mid rectum are essentially a mid-line structure. The upper rectum bends slightly to the left. The recto sigmoid junction usually turns sharply to the right and ventrally. Passing the scope around the recto sigmoid turn may be quite uncomfortable for the patient or even impossible.

The first valve of Houston is seen at 7cm on the left side and the middle valve at 9-11 cm on the right side, which corresponds with the reflection of peritoneum of the middle third of the rectum. At about 15 cm particularly on the left side, the pulsation of common iliac artery is visible. At this level, the scope will be pointing towards the umbilicus once again. It is important to pull back the instrument from time to time "standoff" the bowel wall and reassess the direction of the lumen ahead. Prolonged 'Slide by' is contra indicated. Whilst it is desirable to pass the Sigmoidoscope to its full length, indication for this would be assessed in the light of the patient's symptoms and the degree of discomfort.

14.2. It is on withdrawal, the most attention is given for the pathology. Excessive inflation with air should be avoided. The scope is withdrawn in zigzag fashion so that the lumen is kept in view always. Biopsy of the suspected lesions should be done. But the biopsy should be the last step in the sigmoidoscopy as the biopsy may cause certain amount of bleeding, which obscures subsequent view. Before removing the scope, air in the rectum must be released by removing the eye piece of the scope.

15. RECORDING THE FINDINGS

The findings of inspection, rectal examination, proctscopy, and sigmoidoscopy should be clearly recorded. In rectal examination when a growth is made out, a complete description of the growth should be recorded. The nature of the lesion either ulcerative, proliferative or ulceroproliferative, involvement of the rectal wall, consistency, lower limit in relation to dentate line, upper limit could be reached or not, involvement of muscle layer and extra rectal plane, whether biopsy was done or not. It is advisable to do biopsy in the first examination itself. These recording are valuable to decide the type and scope of operation and other forms of treatment for the patient.

16. GENERAL MEDICAL HISTORY REGARDING

Cardiopulmonary, Vascular, diabetes, renal function should be elicited and recorded.

CHAPTER 2

ANO RECTAL TRAUMA

Traumatic injuries to the anus and anal sphincters are rare. Abundant ischiorectal and gluteal soft tissues generally protect the sphincters except most severe of traumatic injuries. The abundant blood supply to this region promotes healing and diminishes the risk of tissue necrosis. When traumatic forces are strong enough, the Perianal injury may also extensive, that the anus can be separated from the surrounding tissues. The most common cause of injury to anorectal region is iatrogenic. Iatrogenic injury is most often identified at the time of surgery and to be corrected accordingly This includes obstetrical injury as well as anorectal procedures.

1. TRAUMATIC INJURY

1.1. Traumatic injury may be caused by

i. impalement (Pierce with sharp instrument).
ii. Straddle Injury (Standing with legs apart).
iii. Blast injury.
iv. Gunshot injury.
v. First sexual act.
vi. Road traffic accident.
vii. Fall from a height.

1.2. Blunt trauma to the perineum can results in extensive tissue loss and even disruption of the levator ani sling. Associated pelvic fracture can contribute the anal canal and anal sphincter injury.

1.3. Anorectal procedures
Partial anal sphincterotomy, anal fistula surgery, may result in minor degree of incontinence when some amount of division of sphincter, especially in the anterior aspect. Anal dilatation for the treatment of various anorectal disorders results in varying degrees of anal incontinence. Trans anal stapling procedures may cause a fragmentation injury to the internal sphincter.

1.4. Vaginal delivery
The most common cause for the anal sphincter injury is Perianal tear. Laceration of the anal sphincter or anal canal may be the result of deep tear or an extensive episiotomy.

Factors associated with an increased risk of injury:

a. High birth weight baby.
b. Prime gravida.
c. Previous Perianal tear.
d. Instrumentation like delivery forceps, and Vacuum extraction.

1.5. Anorectal foreign body
Anorectal foreign bodies can either be ingested orally or inserted per anum. Although the majority of foreign bodies are inserted for autoerotic purpose, they might have been placed iatrogenically or as a result of assault or trauma. Iatrogenic foreign bodies include rectal thermometer, enema tip, and catheter. The objects placed as the result of assault, trauma, or autoerotism represent a number of diverse collections.

5. Sexual act. Forceful anal intercourse.

2. EVALUATION

In traumatic patients, the initial evaluation should be on the primary Survey of the patient as a whole. Once all life-threading injuries are attended to, a secondary survey to be done for other injuries including the perineum and external genitalia.

2.1. In acute traumatic situation
The Perianal injury is usually fairly evidence, but the sphincter injury to be assessed. Digital rectal examination is essential in assessing the extend of the injury, sphincter integrity, tone, and contractibility.

2.2. In blunt or penetrating trauma
The initial evaluation should document the extend of soft tissue injury and loss of soft tissue, and the degree of contamination. Assessment of sphincter integrity, mucosal and ano dermal laceration are recorded. Rectal examination and proctoscopy should be done to rule out associated rectal injury. Associated pelvic and Perianal injuries be looked for. This may require a urological and gynaecological evaluation.

2.3. Anal ultra-sonography
CT, Contrast Enhanced CT (CECT), Electromyography (EMG) and manometry are essential in ultimate evaluation of the patient..

3. MANAGEMENT

The initial management is debridement of all devitalized tissue and open drainage of the wound to prevent Perianal sepsis.

In bleeding superficial lacerated wound, the bleeding points are arrested and the lacerated edges are trimmed. Deeper mucosal and ano dermal laceration, particular when they are bleeding, are required suture repair.

3.1. Sphincter Injury

A decision should be made whether or not to perform an immediate repair. Internal sphincter or limited external sphincter injury with minimal loss of tissue, in other wise stable patient, primary sphincter repair may be done. Overlapping Sphincteroplasty is not usually possible and an end to end repair is better in these situations. The anal mucosal wound should be sutured. In patients with acute trauma to the anal sphincter without extensive tissue loss or contamination, immediate repair is a good option.

3.2. In patients with an obvious birth injury, repair should be attempted at the time of injury. A waiting period of 6-12 hours may be required for taking up the patient to operation room where adequate light, instruments, and assistants are available.

For patients with delayed presentation, or the initial repair has failed, waiting for at least 3 mouths till the inflammation and oedema has subsided. This also allows time to assess functional and Psychological assessments if necessary.

3.3. Diverting Stoma

The place of diverting stoma and drain depends on the Perianal tissue damage. Stoma is indicated in extensive Perianal injury or rectal injury and when the anus is floating free of surrounding structures. It is easier for the patient to manage a stoma rather than with severe faecal contamination.

4. ANAL SPHINCTER REPAIR

Different operative techniques are available.

i. Overlapping Sphincteroplasty.

ii. End to End repair

iii. Park post anal repair.

4.1. Overlapping Sphincteroplasty

The most effective technique. In elective surgery, ano rectal Physiology laboratory evaluation to help to determine the extent of the sphincter injury and Pudendal nerve damage. This is the procedure of choice in obstetrical injury.

4.1.1. Technique

A curved Perianal incision is made between the anus and vagina. The recto anal septum is separated to the level the anorectal ring. The sphincter ends are identified laterally in the ischiorectal fossae and the dissection is continued to free the sphincter laterally so that the edges maybe over lapped anteriorly over the anus. It is important not to excise the scar tissue, because it will hold the suture for repair. The ends of the sphincter are wrapped around the anus as far as possible so that the resultant anal orifice just allows an examining finger. The repair is done with interrupted horizontal mattress sutures with non absorbable mono filament suture material.

Anterior Levator plasty may be performed at the time of sphincter repair to further lengthen the anal canal. The Perianal body should be reconstructed and the soft tissues are approximated. Skin edges are closed. The reconstruction of Perianal body results in a greater increase the distance between the anus and vaginal introitus. The success of this technique depends on:

i. Adequate residual muscle mass.

ii. The intact neuron muscular bundles.

iii. Retaining the scar tissue around the muscle ends.

5. MUSCLE TRANSPOSITION

Due to extensive injury to the sphincters, perineum, or the pelvic floor, or the pudendal nerve damage, it may not be possible to reconstruct the anal sphincters. In this situation, transposition of either the gluteal muscle or gracilis Muscle may be a better option. Transposition is made to fill a large soft tissue defect or for actual sphincter reconstruction.

5.1. Gluteal muscle transposition

The dual neurovascular supply is advantage for partial gluteal muscle transposition. In addition, the gluteal muscle function as an accessory muscle in maintaining constipation. Based on the inferior gluteal vessels and nerve supply segment, bilateral flaps of gluteal muscles are taken. Each flab is split equally and passed anterior and posterior to the anal canal from each side and sutured in an overlapping position. The opposing pull from both muscles create an valve like sling around the anus. Because only partial muscle is trans positioned, there is no adverse effect on hip and thigh mobility.

5.2. Gracilis muscle transposition

The gracilis muscles is harvested and wrapped around the anal canal. It may be stimulated or non-stimulated. The stimulated or dynamic Graciloplasty converts a fast twitch muscle into a low twitch muscle capable of sustained activity. This stimulation gives the gracilis muscle the property required to maintain sustained contraction and function as a sphincter.

6. ARTIFICIAL SPHINCTER

Artificial anal sphincter is made based on the principles of artificial urinary sphincter. This device Acticon Neosphincter (American medical system) is the option for and sphincter replacement in those i. Who have failed primary repair. ii. Suffer from concomitant neuropathy. iii. Have lost too much of Sphincter to undergo repair.

The system consists of a cuff that is wrapped around the anal canal just below the top of the anorectal ring, a pressure regulating balloon is placed within the pelvis and a control pump located in the scrotum or labia. The implant procedure is simple comparing the muscle transposition procedure. But the indication for artificial sphincter is definite, where muscle transposition cannot be done.

7. INJURY TO THE LOWER RECTUM

Blood discharge from the anus and a palpable hole in the rectal wall are confirmatory. The management is based on the three basic principles developed in war injury, and is very effective in reducing the morbidity and mortality:

i. Diverting Sigmoid ostomy.
ii. Presacral drainage.
iii. Rectal washout.

The routine use in civil injury has been challenged in recent years. In most civilian injury, the rectal washout have been omitted with no change in outcome result. Colostomy should be created as distally as possible.

8. INJURY TO ANAL CANAL

Haemostasis is obtained and the lacerated margins of the wound are excised while taking care to spare as much sphincter as possible. The wound is often left open. Colostomy is indicated only in very extensive anal and perianal lacerations.

In emergency Sphincter reconstruction, the sutures do not hold well in the traumatised muscle, nerve lesion can result from difficult dissection in a bloody field and all these can lead to failure, which will result in compromising success of further reconstruction.

9. RECTAL FOREIGN BODY

Self-inserted foreign bodies whatever their size and shape do not ordinarily cause rectal injury that goes deeper than the mucosa. When the foreign body is inserted due to sexual assault, perforation of the rectum at the level of peritoneal reflection or even at recto sigmoid junction are not exceptional. Removal of foreign body maybe done through anal canal under local, regional, or general anaesthesia, which prevent muscular disruption due to forceful stretching. Many instruments and manoeuvre to grabbing the foreign body have been described. If there is, difficulty in extraction occurs or the risk of laceration of rectal wall or anal canal, laparotomy may be indicated. The foreign body is pushed down from above to the anus. If it is not possible the upper rectal wall is opened, and the foreign body is extracted from above. A post extraction proctoscopy is mandatory to ensure the integrity of the rectal wall.

CHAPTER 3

FUNCTIONAL ANORECTAL PAIN

Functional anorectal pains are those anorectal pain and pelvic pain disorder in which there is no underlying structural or specific pathology. Based upon the clinical presentation it is classified as:

1. Levator ani syndrome
2. Coccygodynia
3. Proctalgia fugax
4. Chronic idiopathic pain.
5. Post proctectomy syndrome.
6. Pudendal nerve entrapment syndrome.

1. LEVATOR ANI SYNDROME

This is also known as

i. Levator spasm.
ii. Puborectalis syndrome.
iii. Pyriform syndrome.
iv. Pelvic tension myalgia.
v. Diaphragma Pelvic Spastica.

1.1. Prevalence

The Prevalence of this condition in general population is around 6% and is found commonly at 30-60 years of age. The symptoms are attributed to spasm of levator ani muscle, the Pathophysiology of which is not known. Its association with Psychosocial disorder is also not clear.

1.2. Symptoms
The symptoms are characterized by relatively constant or frequent dull anorectal pain, often aggravated by long period of sitting or upright position. The pain is associated with tenderness to palpation of the levator ani muscle without any organic diseases, which can explain the pain.

1.3. Rome III Criteria
i. Chronic or recurrent rectal pain.
ii. Duration of pain more than 20 minutes.
iii. Exclusion of other causes of rectal pain.

These three mandatory criteria preferably with more than 3 month's duration.

1.4. Physical examination
Physical examination may reveal over contracted levator ani muscle with acute tenderness in levator ani muscle on palpation. The tenderness is often asymmetric and more frequently in the left side.

1.5. Diagnosis
The diagnosis is based upon the characteristic symptoms in the absence of anorectal or pelvic pathology. The opportunity of examining the patients during the attack of pain seldom occurs. The patient may complaints of a sudden onset of severe pain either in the anus or in the rectum, or in the perineum and it is usually self-limited. The duration of pain rarely last more than 30 minutes. Pain occurs in the night with spasm and the patients have some relieve of pain by hip flexion. It may be associated with mucus discharge per rectum and sometimes there may be abdominal distension. On rectal examination, the pain may be reproduced by palpating the lateral aspect of the pelvic floor and the pain is relieved by levator massage.

2. COCCYGODYNIA

Coccygodynia is considered as a part of levator ani syndrome. The pain is probably caused by the spasm of the Pubococcygeal part of the levator ani muscle. The pain is directed towards the coccyx and the pain may radiate to gluteal region and thigh.

Classically the pain exacerbates when the patient rises from the sitting position. On palpation there is tenderness on the coccyx rather than in the levator ani muscle.

3. PROCTALGIA FUGAX

Proctalgia Fugax is a condition where there is sudden, severe, intermittent pain in the anal region lasting for several seconds or minutes in the absence of any organic cause to explain the pain. Occasionally the pain may last up to 30 minutes. About 90% of cases the pain is localised to anus and exacerbation occasionally occurs after intercourse. It is significantly more common in patients with irritable bowel syndrome. The pain in Proctalgia Fugax is of considerable severity and it first feels like cramp or spasm is the rectum 5-10 cms above the anal verge. It gradually increases in intensity till it become unbearable and sometimes causes fainting. After reaching a peak it gradually subsides. The symptoms are worst in the night. The pain is precipitated by anxiety or stressful condition. It is suggested that the pain is due to spasm of levator ani muscle. The pain has been described as cramping, stabbing and may range from uncomfortable to unbearable and radiating. The symptom rarely occurs before puberty and both sexes are affected equally. The pain occurs infrequently, once in a month or less often. Hereditary form of the disease is also reported where there is associated hypertrophy of the internal anal sphincter. During the episode of pain there is increased myoelectrical activity and anal resting pressure.

3.1. Clinical examination
These patients may have genuine fear of malignancy, sexually transmitted diseases etc. Therefore, a thorough clinical examination should be done

including neurological examination, particularly lumbosacral region. Functional assessment of anal Sphincter and Pelvic Floor Muscles to be done. Proctoscopy and sigmoidoscopy are essential to exclude any pathology in the anal canal and rectum.

4. CHRONIC IDIOPATHIC ANAL PAIN

In this condition there is characteristic pelvic, Perianal or anorectal pain associated with a feeling of something is obstructing in the rectum. Female patients often describe the pain as bearing down discomfort, like a labour pain or feeling of something often described as a ball obstructing in the ano rectum. There may be tenismus in some cases. The discomfort or pain usually maximal when standing still and is released by lying down. About 50% of patients give history of previous pelvic and anal surgery.

5. POST PROCTECTOMY SYNDROME

This syndrome is termed as "Phantom Rectum". Since the symptoms occur after the abdomino Perianal resection and it is akin to "Phantom limb".The patient complains of pain, described as uncomfortable sensation, as if, the rectum and anal canal are still present.

6. PUDENDAL NERVE ENTRAPMENT (PUDENDAL CANAL SYNDROME)

Characteristically this syndrome causes Perianal pain on sitting. Pain may occur in labia, penis depending upon the sex of the patient, and in anus. The pain is reduced or absent on standing since the levator ani muscles becomes tense while standing and take the pressure off the pudendal nerve. It is believed that the pain is due to entrapment and chronic ischemia of the pudendal nerve into fibrous sling under the levator ani muscle. The pudendal nerve entrapment is more common in women with laxed levator (usually after childbirth) Relief of pain may occur following pudendal nerve block or surgical decompression of the fibrous sling in Alcocks canal.

7. MANAGEMENT OF FUNCTIONAL ANORECTAL PAIN

Since the pain episodes are brief and infrequent, the treatment is unpractical and prevention is not possible. So the patient must be reassured. These syndromes are difficult to manage and the clinician must apply patience and sympathy with the patient. One should always remember that although no obvious cause for the symptoms is present, it does not mean that one does not exist. Probably it may be detected in later years with some research work on this condition.

7.1. Psychological disorders

If any, should be treated accordingly. Many of the patients are emotionally labile or psychologically disturbed. There may be a genuine fear of malignancy, sexually transmitted diseases or colitis. The cardinal feature of all these syndromes is that the clinical examination is normal. However a thorough clinical examination should be done. I. Neurological examination, particularly lumbosacral plexus. ii. Pelvic examination. iii. Functional assessment of anal sphincter and pelvic floor muscle. iv. Proctoscopy and Sigmoidoscopy. After thorough history and detailed clinical examination and investigations, the patient must be reassured that there is no serious underlying disease, so that the patients accept that their problems are "a nuisance rather than a disease".

7.2. Constipation

If present, bulky agents or stimulant suppositories may improve the bowel habit and offer some symptomatic improvements. Some patients have a relief of pain by passing flatus or motion or self-introducing the finger into the rectum. Sitz bath may reduce the pain due to reduction in anal pressure. Non-steroidal anti-inflammatory drugs may relieve the pain in some patients. Digital massage of the levator ani muscle gives some relief in those patients with levator ani syndrome.

7.3. Specific therapy with varying success
i. Inhalation of amyl nitrate; Salbutamol.
ii. Sub lingual nitro glycerine.
iii. Sacral nerve stimulation.
iv. Per rectal steroids injection.
v. Local hydrocortisone injection.

7.4. New techniques
i. Ultrasound guided local anaesthetic or alcohol injection.
ii. High voltage electro galvanic stimulation, to induce levator ani muscle fatigue.

8. SURGICAL TREATMENT

If any, undertaken can often make the problem worse. It is true in coccygectomy.

CHAPTER 4

FISSURE IN ANO

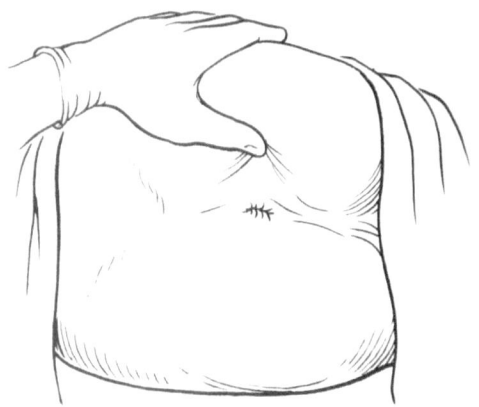

4.01. Inspection. Lift up the buttock

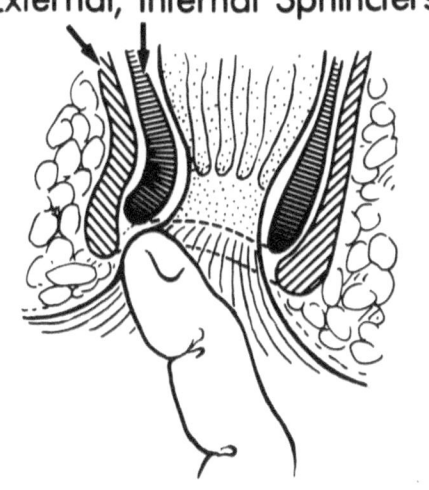

4.02. Inter sphincteric groove

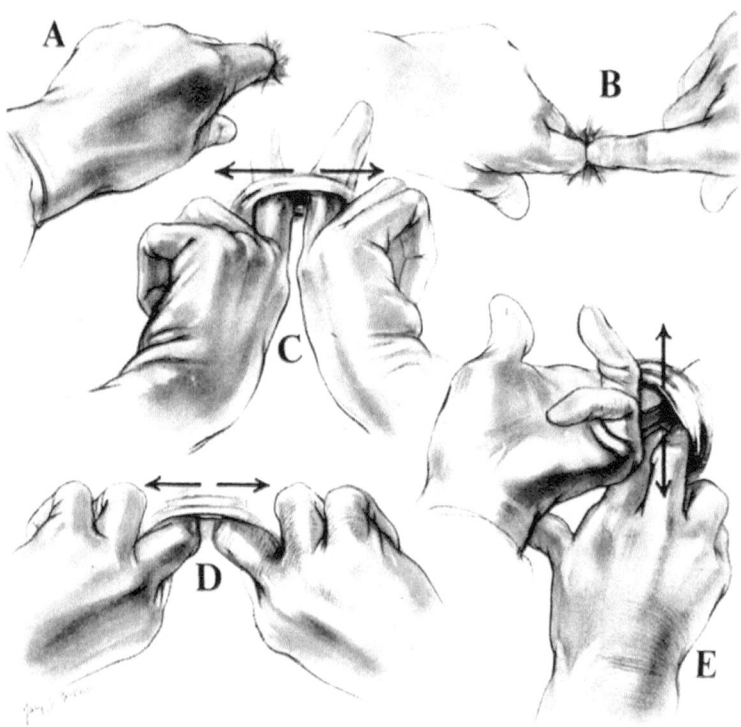

4.03. Steps of Anal dilatation

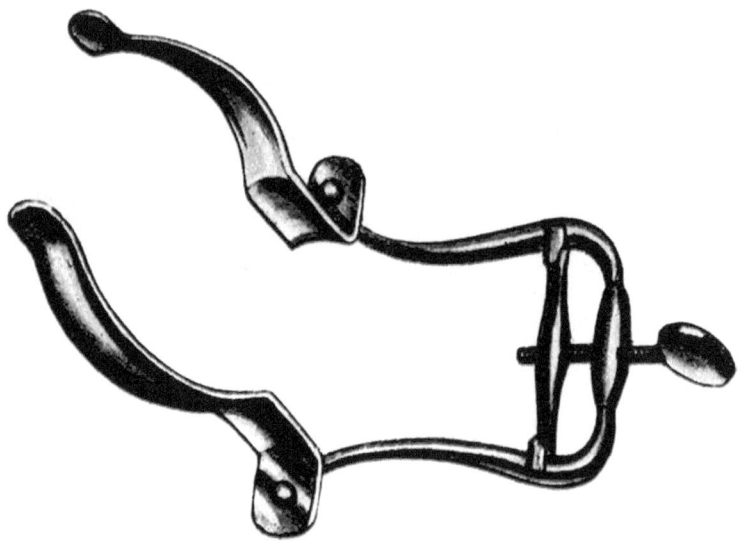

4.04. Park Retractor

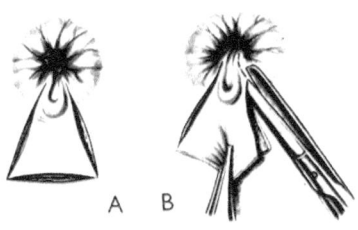
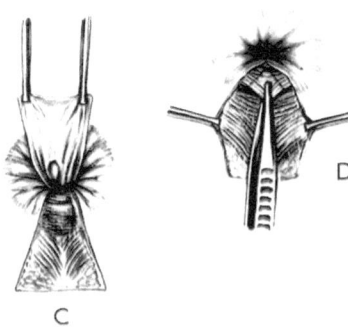

4.05. Excision of anal fissure

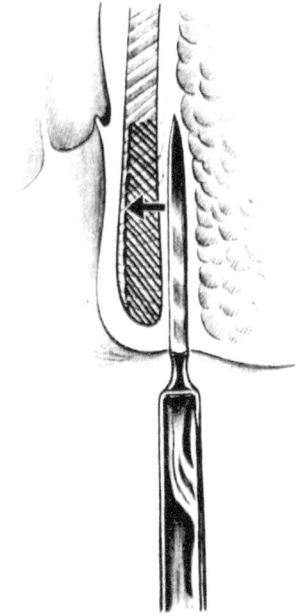

4.06. Lateral subcutaneous sphincterotomy

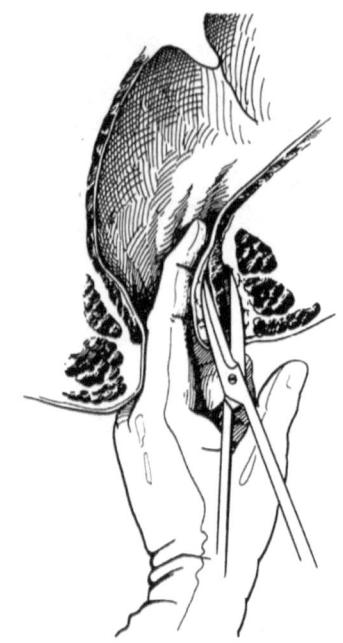

4.07. Sphincterotomy with sharp scissors

Fissure in ano is a longitudinal tear in the distal anal canal extending from the level of dentate line down to the anal verge. This is a common anorectal problem manifesting as pain and bleeding during defecation. The amount of suffering is out of proportion to the size of the lesion. The pathogenesis of anal fissure is still debatable despite of common occurrence.

1. PATHOGENESIS

1.1. The vertical tear in the anoderm between the level of anal verge and anal orifice is superficial to the lower 3rd of internal sphincter. It has no direct relationship to the external sphincter. The Pectin band described by Miles, is the prominent lower edge of internal sphincter.

1.2. Fissures are nearly always single

Consistently occurs in the posterior mid line of the anal verge. Occasionally it occurs in the anterior aspect. In female, a little more likely to have anterior fissure, although posterior position still remains the most common. Postpartum fissures are more frequently anterior, due to the pressure from the foetal head on the relatively unsupported anterior anal canal is the main cause. Previous perianal trauma leads to scaring and tethering of the anal canal leads to more susceptible to trauma in subsequent vaginal delivery.

1.3. Posterior fissure is more common due the following mechanisms

i. The anoderm is more adherent to the underlying tissue in this location and so less mobile.

ii. Posterior angulation of the anal canal.

iii. Elliptical shape of external anal sphincter.

iv. Less perfusion of vascularity in the posterior aspect of anal canal.

1.4. The pain in fissure is due to spasm of internal anal sphincter, which is the continuation of the circular muscle of the rectum. The internal sphincter, therefore, is involuntary muscle. Like colon and rectal muscle, the internal sphincter goes to spasm voluntarily. This voluntary spasm, in response to trauma of the exposed part of the sphincter causes severe pain in the anal fissure. Once the acute fissure developed, internal sphincter undergoes spasm, which is responsible for a vicious circle of the anal pain. Fear of defecation, and passage of hard motion, which further stimulates the internal sphincter activity. Histologically it has been proved that the exposed part of the tissue is those of internal sphincter.

1.5. Previous anal surgery is a contributing factor to the development of fissure. Narrowing of the anal canal may occur as the result of anoderm loss or from persistent internal sphincter muscle spasm. Whatever may be the reason, narrow anal canal is more likely tear with the passage of hard stool.

1.6. A high resting pressure is found in almost all patients with anal fissure. Anal manometry study shows elevation of anal canal pressure. Patients with chronic fissure have an abnormal reflex characterized by an over shooting (Abnormal elevated pressure) of the internal sphincter immediately after relaxation. After treatment of the fissure, the internal sphincter reflex returns to normal and the over shooting phenomenon is absent. A high resting pressure found in chronic anal fissure had been thought to be the consequence rather than the cause. According to this theory a chronic anal fissure is due to the result from non-healing laceration of the anoderm due to constipation.

1.7. Traumatic breakdown in the anoderm normally heals, but patients with pre-existing raised sphincter tone will have impaired micro vascular perfusion of the posterior med line of anoderm and will heal poorly resulting in chronic anal fissure of ischemic origin. This theory is supported by post-mortem angiographic study, showing minimal arterial connections between the terminal branches of bilateral inferior rectal arteries at the posterior aspect of the anus in the midline as well as the demonstration of decrease in anodermal flow at the chronic fissure site.

1.8. Secondary fissure from conditions like Crohn's disease, Tuberculosis, AIDS, Syphilis, Leukaemia, and Anal malignancy should be considered if the fissure presentation is atypical or if the fissure persists despite of conventional therapy.

2. CHRONIC ANAL FISSURE

Chronic anal fissure is most certainly a result of combined effect of hyper tonicity of anal sphincter and deceased anodermal blood flow resulting in ischemic ulcer of the anoderm.

2.1. Local changes in chronic Fissure

2.1.1 Sentinel piles
This is the swelling of the skin at the distal end of the fissure actually at the level of the anal orifice so that it forms a tag like swelling, the so-called sentinel piles. This presumably due to low grade infection

and lymph stasis (oedema). The skin tag has inflamed and oedematous appearance. Later it may undergo fibrosis and persist as permanent skin tag even after the fissure heals.

2.1.2. Hypertrophied anal papilla
The anal valve immediately above the fissure is swollen due to subclinical infection resulting in oedema and later fibrosed and forms the Hypertrophied anal papilla.

2.1.3. In long standing cases of fissure, the lateral edges of the fissure form fibrous in duration

2.1.4. Changes in the Sphincters
The fissure lies in the subcutaneous portion of the anal lining between the level of anal valve and the anal orifice. This portion is situated superficial to the lower most quarter or one third of internal sphincter. Initially the fissure is separated from the sphincter by a thin layer of longitudinal muscle spread over the inner side of the fissure. But eventually the fissure deepens down to the internal sphincter so as to expose the circular fibres of the internal sphincter in the floor of the fissure. At no stage, the external sphincter has direct relation to the fissure. The structure identified as Pectin Band, is the prominent lower edge of the internal sphincter. When the sphincter fibres are exposed, the sphincter goes for tight spasm. This increased sphincter tone is demonstrated by rectal manometry study. The anorectal manometry study also shows increased maximum anal resting pressure (MARP) in patients with chronic anal fissure.

3. PAIN

Like involuntary muscle of colon and rectum, the internal sphincter, which is the continuation of the circular, muscle of the rectum possess the ability to go into spasm involuntarily. It is primarily this involuntary spasm of the internal sphincter is responsible for the pain in the anal fissure. In relatively recent fissure sometimes, require surgery because of the severity of the pain, which the patient is unwilling to tolerate any longer.

4. FISTULA

Frank suppuration may occur is the floor of the fissure, which extends into the surrounding tissue to form a perianal abscess, which may discharge into the anal canal or may burst externally to produce a low anal fistula. Spasm of the internal sphincter brings the lateral edges of the fissure together so that the discharge from the crack is damped back or pocketed and healing by granulation tissue from depth cannot take place. Usually the external opening of the fistula lies close to the midline a short distance behind the anus.

5. CLINICAL PRESENTATION

In majority of cases, constipation is the precipitating factor for the fissure. Diarrhoea can also cause fissure in some cases particularly in elderly persons. Fissures are more common in young childhood and middle age. Both sexes are equally affected. In male, it is nearly always posterior midline. Females are a little more likely to have anterior fissure, although posterior fissure remains more common. Pain may be severe and long lasting. The patients describe the pain as sharp, spearing, burring, Knife like pain associated with passage of stool and lasting for a variable length of time, it may last for just a moment or as long as an hour. In some patients the pain is so severe that they are frighten to pass motion and they may prefer to remain in a constipated state. The pain may be severe enough to interfere with micturition.

Bleeding associated with fissure is always bright red and frequently occurs after motion. Sometimes the motion may have streak of blood or blood lining. There may be discharge, swelling in the anal margin area, and itching around the anus.

6. DIAGNOSIS

Based up on the history the diagnosis of the anal fissure can usually made with a high degree of accuracy. Anal fissure can be seen well by applying gentle traction at the buttocks (fig7.01) and inter sphincteric groove can be seen easily (fig7.02)

6.1. Rectal examination

Though some surgeons are against doing rectal examinations in acute fissures, it is better to do rectal examination to exclude any serious pathology in the anus, and to give direction for the application of medications like local anaesthetic gel. As the patients are very apprehensive for the rectal examination, gentleness must be adapted while doing the rectal examination. Anaesthetic jelly by the gloved finger is applied into the anoderm and wait for 2-3 minutes. It will help for digital examination and use of small size anoscope for the exclusion of any other pathology within distal rectum and anus. Rectal examination may be facilitated by administration of 3-5 mg of Glycerine Trinitrate sublingually 1-2 minutes before the examination.

6.2. Primary Fissure involves only the anoderm bellow the dentate line. If it extends more proximally, it is almost certain that it is secondary to some other disorder. A primary fissure is usually less than 1cm in length and overlies only the lower third of internal sphincter.

6.3. Fissures with atypical appearance may be secondary to Tuberculosis, inflammatory bowel diseases, venereal diseases, Squamous cell carcinoma. Fissures due to tuberculosis and venereal disease may not be associated with anal sphincter spasm and so there may not be much pain. Tuberculous fissures are multiple with classical undermining edges. Destruction of the sphincter muscle may result in multiple fissures. If the fissure is ectopic or broad base the associated inflammatory bowel disease, Crohn's should be considered.

6.4. External examination to rule out abscess, thrombosis or prolapsed haemorrhoid and other causes of severe anal pain.

7. TREATMENT

7. I. Conservative treatment

The goal of conservative treatment is to try to reduce the pain and break the cycle of the pain.

7.1.1. Avoid constipation

The most important aspect of conservative treatment is avoiding constipation. Hard faecal mass passing through the anal orifice produces repeated anal trauma. Constipation can be avoided by taking large quality of fluids (2 litres/day), more vegetables, banana and seasonal fruits. Milled laxative may be useful in acute stage. Bulk laxative, fibre supplement, Sitz bath and topical medications are advised.

7.1.2. Anaesthetic ointments

To lessening the pain of the fissure and relieve the anal sphincter spasm, ointments or jelly containing anaesthetic agent may be applied locally. Lignocaine jelly relieves the pain within 2-3 minutes. The gloved finger well smeared with lignocaine jelly is introduced in to the anal canal and not smeared on the perianal skin. The best time to apply local ointment or jelly is probably after the motion has passed, but it can be applied even before the defecation or other times as required.

7.1.3. Topical glyceryl Trinitrate

Chemical Sphincterotomy. Nitric oxide has been demonstrated to be an important inhibitory to neurotransmitters to the internal anal sphincter. Therefore the nitric oxide donor tri nitrate has been used. Glyceryl tri nitrate when applied locally, temporarily reduces the internal sphincter tone and there by reduces the maximal anal pressure. This clinical sphincterotomy without causing permanent damage to the anal sphincter mechanisms is being adopted in many centres. Topical glyceryl tri nitrate in 0.2% ointment, applied twice a day to the anoderm, heals the fissure in 60-70% within 8 weeks.

Headache and tachycardia can occur. It is contra indicated in concomitant use of sildenafil (Viagra) because of risk of malignant cardiac arrhythmias.

7.1.4. Calcium channel blocker (DILTIAZEM)

A calcium channel blocker 2% gel is applied to the distal anal canal twice a day reduces the resting pressure significantly and about 50% of acute fissure heals within 8 weeks of therapy. The incidence of headache is less but local irritation may occur.

7.1.5. Phospho diesterase inhibitor

Sildenafil (Viagra). One of the noted side effects of Viagra is that it causes relaxation of internal anal sphincter. Clinical trial is on progress.

7.1.6. Botulinum Toxin(BOTOX)

Injection of Botox inhibits the release of Acetylcholine and thereby causes paresis of the striated muscles. Injection of 10-20 units of Botulinum toxin A (Suspended in I ml of 0.9% Sodium chloride) directly into the internal anal sphincter muscle on each side, total amount 20-40 Units. 80-85% chances of curing the fissure within 6-12 weeks. Some patients may need one more injection. It is more expensive.

8. SURGICAL TREATMENTS

Many surgical procedures have been described, most of which involves destructions of the internal anal sphincter resulting in correction of the sphincter spasm and fibrosis of the internal anal sphincter muscle. This can be achieved by stretching, or partial division of the internal sphincter. Excision of fissure to provide a wide external wound in which the discharge cannot pocket.

Indications for Surgical treatment.
i. Chronic fissure with a large sentinel skin tag.
ii. Indurations on the edges of the fissure.

iii. Exposure of internal anal sphincter fibres.

iv. Abscess or fistula formation.

v. Intolerable pain.

8.1. Stretching of the anal sphincter:

This procedure is simple, and no special sterile instrument is required. The principle of this procedure is careful dilatation of the anal canal and lower rectum under anaesthesia with good muscle relaxant. (fig7.03) The anus is forcefully stretched by introducing first both index fingers and then index and middle fingers of both hands which maintained for 1-2 minutes. During this manoeuvre, the forearms are fully pronated. As the result of stretching, the fissure itself torn more widely open and the fissure heals generally. Early and complete relief of pain is achieved a day or two of the procedure. Usually some sphincter fibres are torn and therefore there may the some extravasations of blood leading to Perianal bruising.

Some surgeons use Park anal retractor (fig7.04) for dilatation. The retractor is introduced into the anal canal, opened to 4.8 cm, and left in place for 5 minutes. Some use a 40 mm Balloon for dilatation instead of Park retractor.

Results. As per functional result is concerned slight imperfect control of flatus in 12%, faeces in 2% and 20% had noticed unaccountable soiling of the under cloth for some times. The evidence of incontinence varies considerably and depends upon the extend of the dilatation as well as risk factors such as old age, previous vaginal delivery, previous anal operation and neurological diseases. Anal dilatation should be avoided in 3rd degree haemorrhoids as it may cause prolapse of the haemorrhoids. There is moderate reduction in anal sphincter pressure after anal stretching, but it returns to normal during the course of a week after dilatation.

8.2. Excision of anal fissure

This operation was popularized by Gabriel(fig7.05). The fissure is excised with a broad triangular Perianal skin. Internal sphincterotomy is done through the large triangular wound. It may take 4-6 weeks for the wound to heal. Keyhole deformity in the anal region may occur in some cases.

8.3. Sphincterotomy

8.3.1. Posterior sphincterotomy

Posterior midline sphincterotomy is division of internal sphincter from its distal aspects up to the level of dentate line under direct vision. Excision of the indurated fibrous tissue, hypertrophied anal papilla, and sentinel skin tag maybe combined if necessary. The resultant defect when heals, there may be residual posterior mid line defect in the anal canal which is known as' keyhole' deformity of the anal canal. This can cause spillage and difficulty with continence for flatus and sometimes for the faeces.

8.3.2. Lateral subcutaneous sphincterotomy

The procedure is done under local anaesthesia. A bivalve speculum is introduced in the anal canal and gently opened to expose the left lateral wall of the anal canal and now the lower margin of the internal sphincter can be easily palpable. Van Graefe knife is introduced on the outer side of the sphincter lower border through the Perianal skin. The knife is pushed lateral to the lower edge of the internal sphincter and passed vertically upwards in the intersphinteric plane till it lies at the level of the pectinate line. The lower half of the internal sphincter is divided with the knife in the directions of the anal canal(fig7.06).Care should be taken to avoid injury to the lining of the anal canal. To avoid the mucosal injury the inner fibres of the sphincter are ruptured by lateral pressure with finger. The pressure is maintained for few minutes. Associated skin tag and hypertrophied anal papilla can be excised, probably just before the sphincterotomy.

8.3.3. Open sphincterotomy

Incision is made on the left lateral aspect of the anal canal exposing the portion of the internal sphincter to be divided. Division of the sphincter is done under direct vision and the wound is left open. Now the technique is modified where the anal canal is not opened. The perianal skin is incised, sub mucosal dissection done and the distal internal sphincter is divided.

8.3.4. Notaras Technique

A narrow blade scalpel is introduced through the perianal skin and pushed in cephalic direction with the blade is between the anoderm and the internal sphincter. When the tip of the blade reached the dentate line, the blade is tuned outwards and the internal sphincter is divided. Some surgeons use narrow pointed scissors instead of knife(fig7.07).

All fibres of the distal internal sphincter muscle must be divided because any residual film will go into intense spasm to compensate the divided sphincter. Proximal one third of the sphincter must be left intact to maintain continence.

8.3.5. Bilateral internal sphincterotomy

It is indicated in chronic anal fissure developing in the scar from previous Anorectal surgery. Incisions are made at left lateral and rights lateral position in the internal sphincter. It may be more effectively release the stenotic distal intersphinteric ridge. As long the proximal internal sphincter is left, no significant incontinence occurs.

8.3.6. Laser treatment

Portable laser equipment is available for the treatment of fissure. By the use of laser, the anal fissure is vaporized. This is the recent technique to treat the anal fissures.

6.3.7. Ano plasty

Ano plasty permits excision of the fissure and widening out of the anal canal. Various methods of ano plasty are described. When there is a true loss of anoderm, advancement flap may be more useful. Patients with low maximal anal resting pressure V-Y ano plasty or an island advancement flap is more desirable.

9. POST-OPERATIVE CARE

Bulk Laxative and Sitz Bath are routinely recommended. The best anal dilator is a well formed mouldable stool. If the normal dilatation is obviated, by laxative or enema gradual anal stenosis may occur.

10. ATYPICAL ANAL FISSURES

Fissures due to inflammatory bowel disease, may be the mucosal manifestations of the disease and this is no internal sphincter spasm. So in these cases anal dilatation or sphincterotomy is not indicated. Fissures in Crohn's disease are multiple, asymptomatic, and may associated with anal stenosis and with prominent skin tags. Fissures in Crohn's disease heal during medical treatment. If it is associated with anal stenosis only minimal anal dilatation should be done.

Fissures of tuberculus origin needs full course of anti tuberculus treatment. Fissures due to specific causes to be treated accordingly.

CHAPTER 5

HAEMORRHOIDS

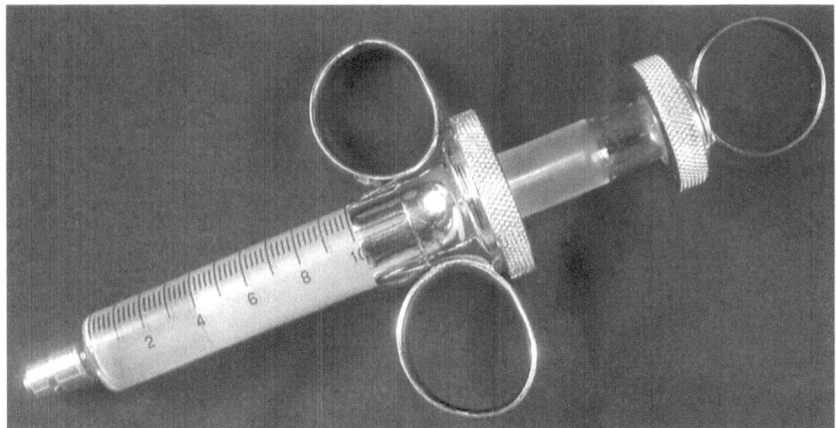

5.01. Gabriel's syringe

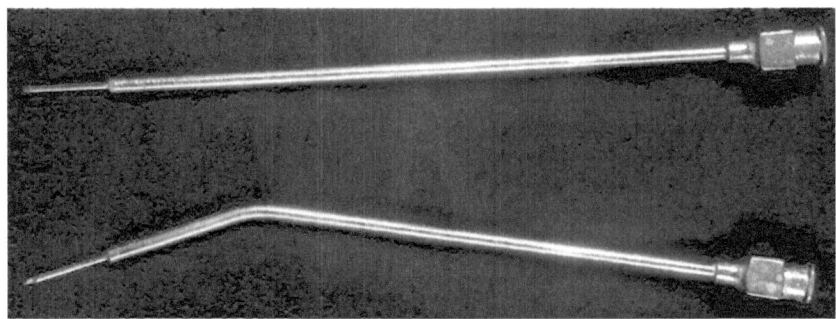

5.02. Needle for injection

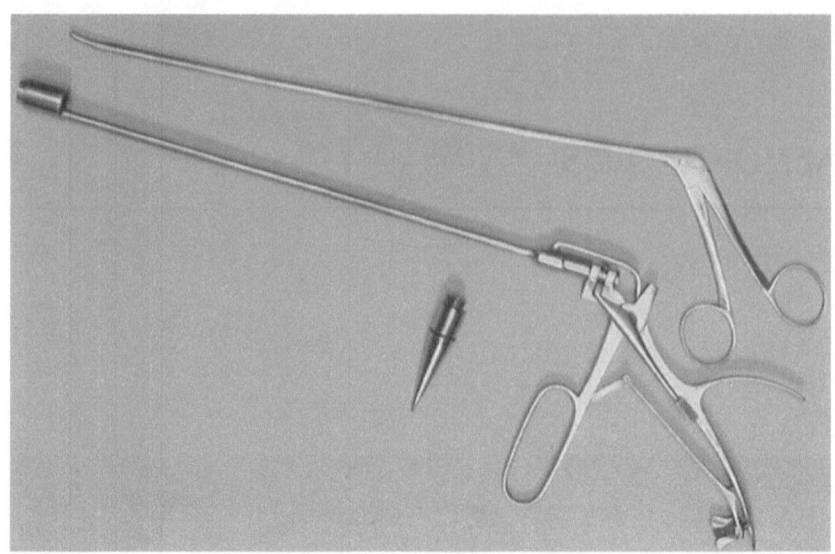

5. 03. Rubber band ligator

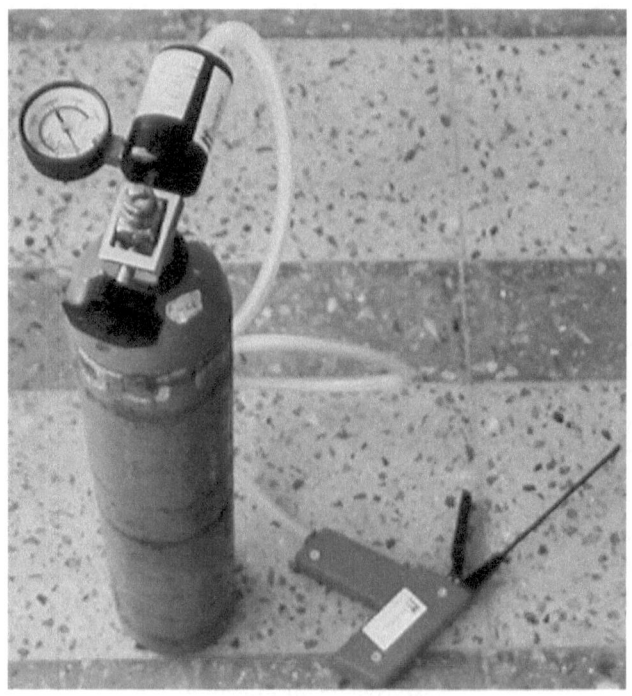

5.04. Cryo apparatus

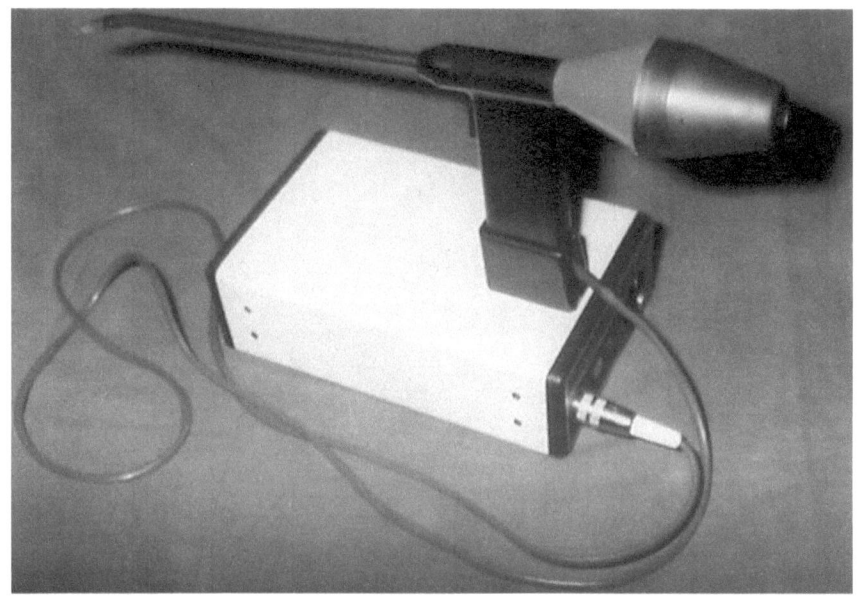

5.05. Infra-Red Coagulator

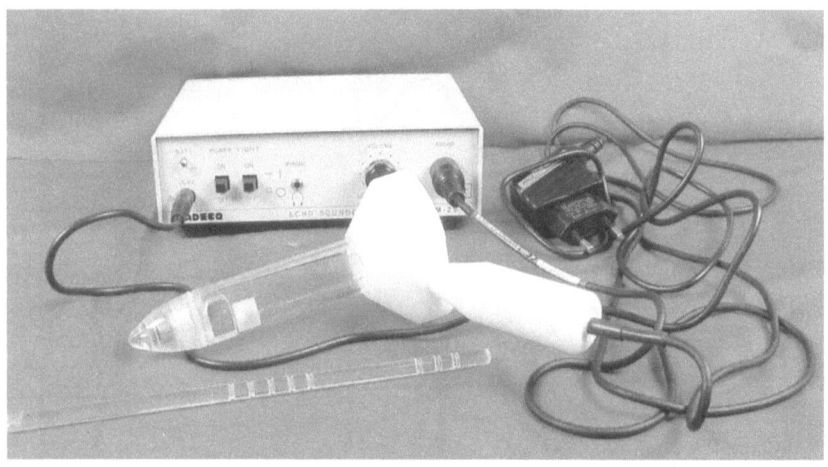

5.06. Doppler Guided Haemorrhoidal artery Ligator

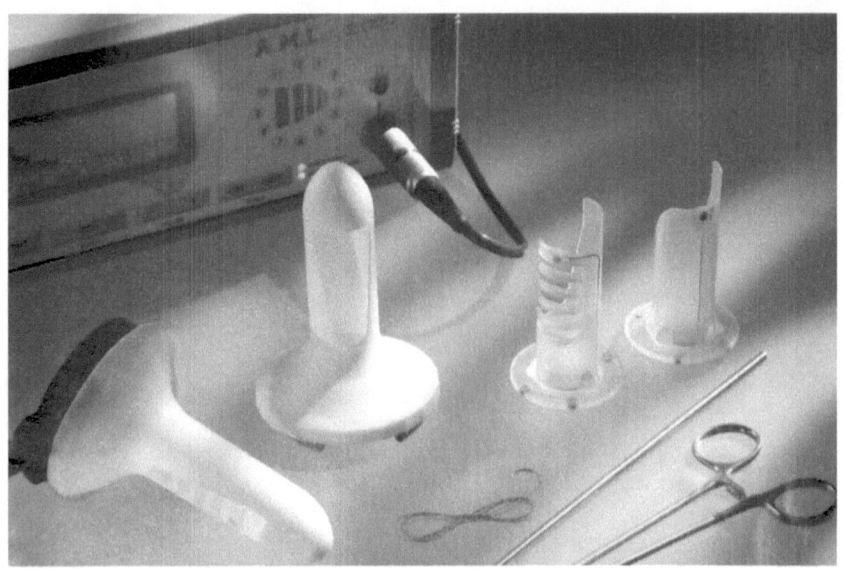

5.07. Hemorrhoidopexy equipment

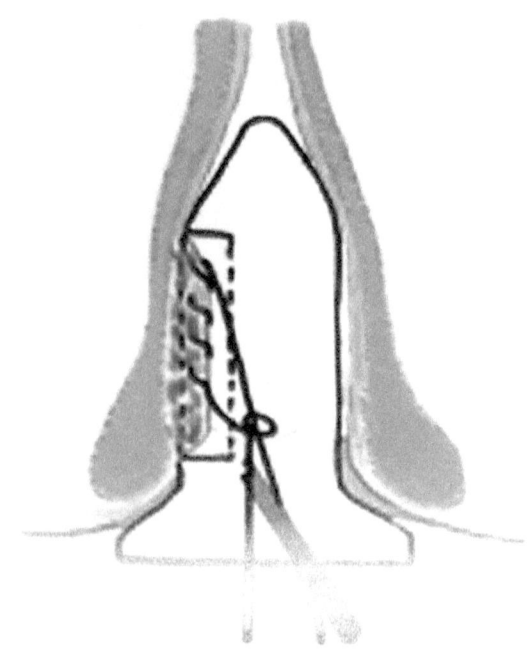

5.08. Procedure

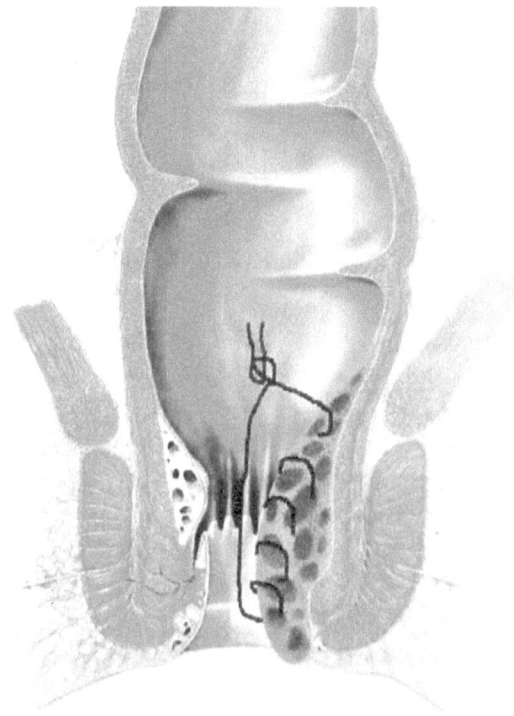

5.09. Final step

Haemorrhoids are one of the commonest ailments that affect the humanity. The exact prevalence of haemorrhoids is difficult to estimate. Patients attribute nearly all complaints in or near the rectum to haemorrhoids. Therefore the ultimate diagnosis and management truly must rest with an experienced clinician.

1. DEFINITION

The word" haemorrhoid" is derived from the Greek words haem (Blood.) and rhoos (Flowing) meaning flowing of blood. The word ' Piles' means Pile or a ball. So we should call this disease as piles when the patient complaints of swelling and haemorrhoid when the presenting symptom is bleeding.

2. CORPUS CAVERNOSUM

The rich plexus of vascular tissue under lower rectal mucosa and anal canal is called corpus cavernosum recti, which connects arteries and veins without intervening capillaries. Branches of superior, middle and inferior rectal vessels feed this plexus. There are three main anal cushions located in left lateral, right anterior and right posterior position corresponding to branches of superior rectal vessels. This is better identify these cushions like this than describing their position as 3,7, and 11 o'clock.

2.1. Functions of Corpus Cavernosum

i. The vascular cushion have physiological role in maintaining the continence as the cushion act like a" washer" effect that allows complete closure of the rectal lumen which cannot be achieved by the muscular tube alone.

ii. These cushions also provide a comprehensive protective lining of the under lying anal sphincter.

iii. The anal cushions also involved in the anorectal inhibitory reflex. Small amount of rectal distension initiates relaxation of internal sphincter followed by contraction of the external sphincter this allows a small quantity of rectal content to enter into the lower rectum and by sampling mechanism, the anorectal junction distinguishes between solid, liquid, and gas, and adjust the continence accordingly.

iv. The anal cushions contribute 15-20 % of anal resting pressure.

3. PATHOGENESIS OF HAEMORRHOIDS

3.1. Traditionally internal haemorrhoids have been regarded as essentially varicosity of the venous plexus in the wall of the anal canal and the lower most centimetres or so of the rectum. These veins are radicals of superior haemorrhoidal vein. The contents of haemorrhoids are venous plexus, a small arterial twig that is one of the ultimate branches of the superior haemorrhoidal artery, and certain amount of loose sub mucosa and areola tissues surrounding the vessels. In long standing haemorrhoids, the areola tissue is converted into dense fibrous tissue and the haemorrhoids become palpable.

3.2. According to Thomson, the sub mucosa does not form continuous ring in the anal canal and it is a discontinued series of vascular cushion, which contributes the left lateral, and right anterior and posterior position. The sub mucosal layer of these cushions is rich in blood vessels and muscular fibres called muscularis sub mucosa ani. These muscular fibres arise from internal anal sphincter and the conjoined longitudinal muscle fibres are responsible for maintaining the adhesions of the mucosa and sub mucosal tissues to the internal sphincter and blood vessels of the sub mucosa. The longitudinal muscle of the rectum gives anchoring muscular extension to the internal anal sphincter and the anal cushions(ligament of Treitz) by keeping them in position and allow them to function normally. The muscle changes with age showing an increase in the amount of connective tissue this leads to loss in elasticity, allowing anchoring muscle fibres that gives support to the anal cushion and sphincter complex to fragments resulting in potential prolapse of haemorrhoidal tissue. Therefore, the development of Haemorrhoids from the anal cushion may be seen as a natural progression of the ageing progress. The haemorrhoidal veins in the sub mucosa of the anal canal are firmly supported by the close apposition of the walls of the anal canal by the contraction of the sphincter. During defecation, the pressure in the portal system is increased by straining; distension of the haemorrhoidal veins is liable to occur. Descending mass of faeces, especially, when the motion is hard and constipated or constriction of the veins by the contracting rectal muscle the haemorrhoid vessels dilate.

3.3. Some Authors are of opinion that the swollen tissue of ano rectum might represent" corpus cavernosum recti" and they have demonstrated numerous arterio venues communication in the anal region.

3.4. Idiopathic haemorrhoids are commonly seen in practice. Members of a family including children are affected. It may be due to some structural weakness of the wall of the haemorrhoidal veins. Varicose veins of the leg and Haemorrhoids are seen in same persons suggesting more wide spread defect of the venous system.

3.5. There is some degree of distension of the haemorrhoidal venous plexus in the anal canal during the act of defecation. In constipation, the patient has to strain repeatedly and for a prolonged time. So there is marked distension effect on the haemorrhoidal plexus and resulting in haemorrhoid formation in due course. Spending long time sitting on the toilet, with unsupported and relaxed perineum leads to engorgement of the anal cushion and increases the downward shearing force upon them but in fact, it should be pulled upwards during defecation.

3.6. Haemorrhoids in pregnancy. In pregnancy there is increased vascularity and enlarged uterus obstructing the free flow of the venous return resulting in haemorrhoids formation. The external haemorrhoids also become engorged. A haemorrhoid during pregnancy regresses after delivery. When the external haemorrhoids regress lead to redundancy of the perianal skin.

3.7. Carcinoma of middle third of rectum may obstruct the superior haemorrhoidal vein and may lead to engorgement of haemorrhoid plexus. These patients may present as haemorrhoids and proper rectal examination, proctoscopy, sigmoidoscopy reveal the cancer.

3.8. Haemorrhoids are not caused by heavy work or exertion. No occupational group seems specially proves the cause of haemorrhoids.

3.9. Portal hypertension causes rectal varices and the bleeding from these varices is profuse and dark, whereas the bleeding from haemorrhoids is bright red.

4. CLASSIFICATION OF HAEMORRHOIDS

The haemorrhoids are clarified as:

i. Vascular haemorrhoids.
ii. Mucosal haemorrhoids.

iii. Internal haemorrhoids.

iv. External haemorrhoids.

4.1. Vascular haemorrhoids

It is seen mainly in young individuals. The presenting symptom is bleeding per rectum.

4.2. Mucosal haemorrhoids

Seen more often in old patients, which are formed by large thickened mucosa. The main presenting symptoms are, a feeling of some short of obstruction during the initial act of defecation and a sense of incomplete evacuation.

4.3. Internal haemorrhoids

It is due to the redundant part of mucous member of the rectum and anal canal above the dentate line. Depending upon the symptoms and the extend of the prolapse, internal haemorrhoids are classified as:

i. First degree. Which bleeds.

ii. Second degree. Bleeds, prolapse and reduced spontaneously.

iii. Third degree. Bleeds, prolapse, and required manual reduction.

iv. Fourth degree. Bleeds, incarcerated, and cannot be reduced.

4.4. External haemorrhoids

They occur in the perianal region. They are situated below the dentate line and are covered by anoderm. The anal skin tags are the result of previous attacks of external haemorrhoids.

5. SYMPTOMS

The main symptoms of haemorrhoids are bleeding, protrusion, pain, discharge, and irritation.

5.1. Bleeding

The most common symptom is bleeding. Initially there is a slight streak of blood on constipated motion. Later, drips of blood for a minute after the motion has passed. When the haemorrhoid prolapsed it becomes congested and bleeding can occur apart from defecation at any time and spontaneous bleeding may occur. The blood is bright red in colour and therefore, the bleeding is from arterial rather than venous source. The blood loss may be occasional or severe and persistent enough to cause anaemia. In massive bleeding, the patient may have an urgent desire to defecate and a loose motion is passed along with blood. The volume of the blood may be considerable but stops quickly.

5.2. Protrusion

Initially the protrusions occur during defecation and get reduced spontaneously after the act. Later the protrusion occurs during defecation and the patient has to push into the anal canal after motion. At this stage the prolapse can occur on coughing, sneezing, or passing flatus. In old age it is permanently prolapsed with anal mucosa exposed.

5.3. Pain

Usually haemorrhoids are associated with some anal discomforts. When thrombosis occurs, the pain may be moderate to severe, depending upon the degree of engorgement. Severe pain may be due to associated conditions like, most commonly, fissure or an anal abscess.

5.4. Discharge and irritation

Soiling of the underclothing with mucus may occur when the prolapsed haemorrhoid present. Irritation of perianal skin is present in varying degree of intensity in 3nd degree and 4th degree. However, the typical skin change that occurs in pruritus ani is not common.

5.5. Painful mass in the anal region

When thrombosis of the prolapsed haemorrhoids occurs, the patient may present for a painful mass the anus and this is the most common complication occurs suddenly. Tissue tension rises within and outside the anal canal is the cause for the pain and oedema. The condition can be diagnosed by inspection itself. The natural history of the thrombosed haemorrhoids is one of slow resolution. The oedema and inflammatory swelling reduces in a course of 4-5 days and complete resolution occurs in 4-6 weeks leaving enlarged skin tag.

5.6. Anaemia

Repeated profuse anal bleeding causes iron deficiency anaemia with haemoglobin as low as 45% or even low. In cases of severe anaemia one should always suspect another possible occult cause form intestinal bleeding. It is advised to check the haemoglobin regularly after the haemorrhoid is successfully treated to ensure that the cure of anaemia is permanent.

6. CLINICAL EXAMINATION

A detailed history is very important in the diagnosis of the haemorrhoids. The colour and the character of the anorectal bleeding and the relief obtained from reduction of the prolapsed mass into the anal canal leads to the diagnosis. The presence of haemorrhoid does not exclude other causes of bleeding. Third degree haemorrhoid is a protruding mass, the outer part of which is covered with skin, the inner portion with red or purplish anal mucosa, the junction between the two area being marked by a linear furrow.

6.1. Rectal examination

Usually uncomplicated haemorrhoids are not palpable. Large haemorrhoids can be felt as a soft elevation of the anal canal mucosa just above the dentate line and extends up to the Anorectal ring.

6.2. Proctoscopy

Proctoscopy permits accurate diagnosis of haemorrhoids as well as the degree of prolapse on straining when the proctoscope is being withdrawing.

6.3. Sigmoidoscopy

Sigmoidoscopy is essential to exclude any pathology beyond the reach of the proctoscope. In individuals more than 40years of age with the haemorrhoids, Sigmoidoscopy should be done. one should always keep in mind that other anorectal pathological conditions may present with similar symptoms. They include: i. Rectal prolapse, partial or complete. ii. Polyps. iii. Carcinoma. The patients need a complete colonic evaluations in those who are at the risk, based on the family history and old age. Some patients may present along with the Haemorrhoids, narrowing of the calibre of the anal canal which may probably due to abuse of laxatives.

6.4. Patients with haemorrhoids and associated soiling or incontinence, may require ano rectal Physiology study and endoanal ultra sonogram, as these patient have high risk of developing incontinence after surgery.

7. TREATMENT

The management of haemorrhoids is based on the degree of the vascular cushion, the type, and the severity of the symptoms. Numerous therapeutic modalities have been advocated. The choice of method of treatment is also dependence upon the expertise of the doctor and Equipments availability. The surgeon must decide the optimal treatment on a combination of appliance, anatomical position, and symptoms. The treatment options include dietary modifications, medical treatment, office procedures for early and less symptomatic haemorrhoids and operative intervention. Non-operative treatment gaining wider acceptance. Not all patients with haemorrhoids require active treatment except some dietary modification.

7.1. Dietary and life style modifications

Life style modification plays an important role for the improvement of symptoms in these patients. Neglecting the first urge to defecate, spending prolonged time at toilet and straining are common defecation errors, which needs to be corrected. Increased fibre intake and water intake, reduced straining at stool, and local hygiene are all the integral part of the management of all degrees of haemorrhoids. The patient should be advised to take diet rich in fibres(20-35 g /day). Fibre supplementation(Psyllium, Methyl cellulose, Calcium poly carbophil) has been shown to improve the overall symptoms and bleeding. Fibre supplementation is usually recommended for the patients who are not taking sufficient fibres intake. Psyllium with water adds moisture to stool and thereby reduces constipation. Bulk forming laxatives are more useful.

7.2. Medical treatment
i. The most effective symptomatic relief can be obtained by warm(40° C) Sitz bath for about 15 minutes or ice pack for limited period.
ii. Topical agents such as creams, lotions, suppositories, and local anaesthetic agents have been used, and have been shown to give symptomatic relief.
iii. Calcium Dobesilate can be advised locally as well as systemically. It decreases the capillary permeability, Platelet aggregation, and blood viscosity. Calcium Dobesilate has been found to be safe, fast acting and efficient in treating acute symptoms of haemorrhoids.
iv. Micronized purified Flavonoid fraction acts by enhancing venous tone by prolonging vein wall epinephrine, has been shown to be effective in reducing bleeding from non-prolapsing haemorrhoids.
v. Topical nitric oxide in the form of glyceryl nitrate has been reported effective in strangulated haemorrhoids by decreasing the tone of the internal anal sphincter. Even though topical agents may improve the symptoms, it is unlikely that they will eliminate and ultimately cure the haemorrhoids.

7.3. Non-surgical treatment

7.3.1. Injection therapy (Sclerotherapy)
Mitehell of Clinton pioneered injection therapy in 1871. He kept it secret and sold to quacks just before his death. These quacks who roamed in

the United States and they are well known as" piles doctor". Eventually Andrews of Chicago discovered the secret from one of the quacks and gave it to medical profession in 1879.

Sclerotherapy is indicated in 1st and 2nd degree haemorrhoids. It is contra indicated in thrombosed, prolapsed, ulcerated, infected, and gangrenous haemorrhoids.

The chemical agent used is 5% Phenol in vegetable oil, or quinine, urea hydrochloride, Sodium morrhuate. 5 ml of solution is injected into the interstitial tissue (unlike in varicose vein where sclerocent is injected into the vein). A total of 12-15 ml of solution can be used. The injection is given with Gabriel syringe (fig 8.01) through the proctoscope at the base of the haemorrhoids, just below the ano rectal ring. The Gabriel syringe has two lateral rings on the barrel and a ring at the end of the piston for a secured grips. The needle must be 7-5 cms length with straight or slightly angulated with a shoulder on the needle 2cm from its sharp end (fig 8.02). The amounts of fluid to be injected in each site well depend on the laxity of the sub mucosa. The solution must flow freely. Résistance to flow means wrong placement of the needle.

Following injection the red mucosa turns purple. After an hour or so the fluid gravitates down and causes some soreness. First injection is most effective. Subsequent injections are given when the symptoms reappear. Larger the haemorrhoids, the shorter the duration of remission. Repeat Sclerotherapy is difficult because of fibrosis as the result of previous injection. The injection causes fibrosis is in the sub mucosal areolas plane, and adherence of the mucosa with the muscularis. With injection the degree of prolapse is lessened, bleeding is reduced and often stopped completely. This favourable effect is due to interstitial fibrosis. The injected area feels like an indurated mass for about 2-3 weeks, after that it gradually subside.

Complications of Sclerotherapy include pain, haemorrhage, local sepsis, necrosis, ulceration, portal pyemia, Prostatitis, and haematuria. Pain is due to sclerocent travelling down, or the injection is given lowdown on sensitive area. That is why the patients is kept in bed for few hours with foot end is elevated.

Bleeding can be stopped by pressure with proctoscope or finger. Prostatitis and haematuria occur when the sclerocent is given at right anterior haemorrhoid.

7.3.2. Cryotherapy

The principle of cryotherapy is based on cellular destruction through rapid freezing followed by rapid thawing. The freezing temperature of -60 to -80 Centigrade is achieved by nitrous oxide gas and at -180 centigrade by liquid Nitrogen, can eliminate haemorrhoids by necrotizing the vascular cushion due to thrombosis of micro circulation(fig 8.04). The procedure is associated with profuse foul smelling discharge and irritation. In addition to pain and slow healing, inappropriate use of cryotherapy can cause necrosis of internal anal sphincter, resulting in incontinence and in some cases anal stenosis. Therefore, cryotherapy for haemorrhoids is not advocated in many centres now.

7.3.3. INFRA RED COAGULATION (I.R.C.):

The infra-red coagulation is generated by a Tungsten Halogen Lamp. Gold plated reflector and specially made Polymer tubing facilitate the process(fig 8.05). First it was described by Natti and Popularized by Neiger in1979. The infra-red light penetrates the tissue to a level of approximately 3mm in the sub mucosa in the form of heat energy of 100 degree centigrade. This heat causes active burns, leading to tissue destruction and eventually in scaring. It results in not only the destruction of vascular tissue but also tethering of the haemorrhoids and thus prevents bleeding and prolapses.

The site of application is similar to the area advised for sclerosing agents. An ulcerated area develops over the applied sites after 4-5 days, there can be some mucous discharge and a sensation of fullness in the anal region, and discomfort until complete healing occurs. Repeat application may be needed in some patients after 2 months. Infra-red coagulation is indicated in bleeding haemorrhoids without prolapse or with minimal prolapse.

Complications. Transient discomfort during the application of infra-red coagulation is common. If the pain persists, it is because the site chosen is too close to the dentate line. Bleeding can occur in the 6-8 th post application day and can be managed by bed rest and other symptomatic treatment.

7.3.4. RUBBER BAND LIGATION

It is a simple, in expensive, and one of the most widely adopted outpatient procedure for 2 nd and 3rd degree haemorrhoids. The principle of rubber band ligation is fixing the mucosa with the muscle layer of the rectum by causing ulceration. The band results in ischemic necrosis of the tissue, which slough out in a week, time leaving an ulcer, which heals, by fibrosis resulting in fixation of the mucosa with muscle layer of the rectum.

Barron Rubber Band Ligator
The instrument has a hallow drum, 11 mm in diameter (fig 8.03). The rubber band is placed over the drum by means of loading cone. A second drum moves over the outer surface of the first and pushes the rubber band into position over the haemorrhoids. The two drums are mounted on a handle flitted with a trigger device. The haemorrhoid is drawn into the hallow drum by a forceps specially made for, or long Allis forceps. It must be ensured that the rubber band will not grip sensitive area at dentate line. The trigger is pulled, the outer drum slides over the inner drum and pushes the rubber band off the inner drum on to the point of haemorrhoid level. The forceps is released from the haemorrhoid and the ligator is removed. The ligated haemorrhoid has a polyphoidal appearance with the pedicle grasped by the rubber band.

Different modifications were made in the equipment. One such modified instrument was made by Mc Gown suction ligator. The haemorrhoidal mass is drawn into ligating barrel by section thereby avoiding the use of second hand or assistant.

A disposable syringe like ligator, invented by O' Regan, to simplify the procedure for the surgeon as well as for the patient.

Though multiple haemorrhoid masses can be ligated in a single sitting, majority of surgeons prefer two masses at a time and the third one after 4-6 weeks. About 60-70% of cases respond to rubber band ligation with significant symptomatic relief. A second application may be required in the rest of the patients.

Complications of Rubber Band ligation
i. Pain. Immediate severe pain is due to improper level of application where the Band involves the dentate line. In these cases, by using a cataract blade the rubber band is removed immediately.
ii. Delayed severe pain. A sensation of fullness in the anus and severe pain may occur for about 24-48 hours. This is due to the oedema over the band-applied area extending down to the dentate line. It is best treated by complete bed rest and anti-inflammatory drugs.
iii. Bleeding. Passage of blood with the first bowel moment after the procedure is common. The patients should be instructed accordingly to avoid undue apprehension. Delayed bleeding occurs at about 7-10 days after the rubber band ligation, when the band falls off. If the vessels are not occluded by the time, bleeding occurs. Complete bed rest and reassurance will help the situation.
iv. Rarely perianal sepsis and pelvic sepsis have been reported in immuno-suppressed individual.

7.4. Bipolar diathermy coagulation
This technique is designed to produce distraction, ulceration, and fibrosis by local application of heat. This effects is obtained by Bipolar diathermy, an electric current to generate a coagulation of tissue at the end of cautery tip. Heat does not penetrate as deeply as mono polar

coagulation. In each haemorrhoids two second pulse is applied in a suitable location in the same manner as Infra-red coagulation. This can be repeated as many times as required.

LigaSure haemorrhoidectomy – the bipolar electro thermal device is used to excise the haemorrhoidal tissue. The bleeding is less and there is minimal damage to the adjacent tissue.

8. SURGICAL TREATMENT

8.1. Principles in surgical treatment

i.   The single most important factor underlying any surgical treatment of haemorrhoids is, avoid extensive removal of tissue from the anal canal proper.

ii. The anal canal deserves as much respect as urethra or Bile duct.

iii. Surgery that has to be executed in a confined area such as anal canal demands special care, excellent judgment and careful execution.

iv. A stenosis at anal verge or at the level of anorectal ring can be repaired easily, not so with a stenosis of anal canal.

v.   Instruments that stretch the anal canal during surgery should be carefully used.

vi. When the wounds are closed, accurate opposition of margins is most important.

vii. The surgery for haemorrhoids remains the classical operation of Colorectal Speciality and it forms the basis of knowledge and expertise surgery of the anal canal.

viii. When properly learned, haemorrhoidectomy is immensely satisfying the patient, and his family, particularly his wife, and the surgeon because it brings a welcome and permanent cure.

8.2. Haemorrhoids are very common complaint in pregnant women. The symptoms usually resolve after delivery. Conservative treatment is generally preferred. Surgical treatment is only for complicated haemorrhoids.

8.3. Haemorrhoids in HIV patients can be safely managed as in non-infected patients in early stages of the disease. Patients with AIDS, however are at high risk of complications and probably should not undergo surgery except under well controlled circumstances.

8.4. If indicated, haemorrhoidectomy can be safely performed in patients with Ulcerative Colitis in remissions stage, but surgery should be avoided in Crohn's disease. Definitely, any extensive surgical treatment of any anorectal conditions in Inflammatory Bowel disease may result in delayed healing or non-healing of the wound causing greater disability to the patient than before surgery.

8.5. Indications for Surgery
i. Prolapsed haemorrhoids with thrombosis or gangrene.
ii. Ulceration of the haemorrhoids.
iii. Associated lesions like anal Papilla, Fissure and fistula.
iv. Presence of external component.
v. Failure of non-surgical treatment.

Numerous surgical options are available. In conventional procedure, the haemorrhoid mass is excised and either left open to heal by secondary intension (Milligan Morgan haemorrhoidectomy) or closed primarily (Ferguson's haemorrhoidectomy).

Various modifications have come up using different Equipments for excision, like electro cautery, bipolar Coagulation (LigaSure), Harmonial scalpel, circular stapler and Doppler Guided Haemorrhoid Artery Ligation(DGHAL) and DGHAL with Recto Anal Repair(PAR).

8.5.1. Open haemorrhoidectomy (Milligan Morgan)
The choice of anaesthesia and the position of the patient for surgery are individualised and are generally depend on the patient's condition and

surgeon's preference. Milligan Morgan popularised the open technique. Since this procedure is relatively simple it was adopted at one time throughout the world as virtually the only technique up to 1960. Now open haemorrhoidectomy is an option, when the wound cannot be closed, or in the presence of gangrene, or circumferential haemorrhoids. Though the results of open haemorrhoidectomy is excellent there is more pain in the post-operative periods, takes a little longer time to heal, and the post-operative anal stenosis is a little high. The anal stenosis can be avoided by leaving sufficient islands of anoderm between the excised segments.

8.5.2. Closed haemorrhoidectomy (Ferguson)

The closed haemorrhoidectomy has three principle objectives. i. To remove as much vascular tissue as possible without sacrificing anoderm. ii. To minimize post-operative serous discharge by prompt healing with immediate suturing of the anoderm. iii. To prevent anal stenosis that may complicate healing of large raw wound by granulation tissue.

8.5.2.1 Operative technique

After positioning the patient, decision should be made which haemorrhoid should be removed first. Generally, the best defined, lest complex one and that seems to be the most offender should be tackled first. Tissue distortion should be avoided all the time. In larger haemorrhoids, a longer incision should be made with a ratio of 3:1 length to breath. After excision of long triangular segment of haemorrhoidal tissue to the level of Anorectal ring, sufficient undermining of wound edges are made to facilitate the removal of accessory haemorrhoidal tissue and closing the wound. During dissection, damage of the internal sphincter should be avoided. Starting from the pedicle a running suture with 2/0 vicryl is used for the wound closure to co-opt the edges of the wound with minimal tension.

The advantages of closed haemorrhoidectomy:

i. Less post-operative discomfort.
ii. Minimal in patient stay.

iii. Practically no outpatient care of the wound.

iv. No loss of continence.

v. No need for subsequent dilatation.

8.5.2.2. Sub Mucosal Haemorrhoidectomy

This surgery is done by making a linear incision made over the region of the haemorrhoid and then under mining the wound edges carefully, excise the haemorrhoidal tissue without removing the anoderm or skin. The wound is closed with absorbable suture. This Sub mucosal haemorrhoidectomy of Sir Allen Park gave good result in his hand.

8.5.2.3. White Head haemorrhoidectomy

A Circumferential incision is made at the level of the dentate line. Sub mucosal and sub dermal haemorrhoidal tissues are dissected out and excised. The redundant rectal mucosa is excised and the proximal rectal mucosa is sutured circumferentially to the anoderm. The operation is technically difficult, bloody, and with high rate of post-operative stricture. The ectopion is so common that it is called' white head deformity'. Some surgeons, however, claimed good results after modifying the technique.

8.5.2.4. Laser Haemorrhoidectomy

Both Carbon dioxides (CO_2) and Neodymium-Yttrium- Garnet (Nd: YAG) laser have been used in haemorrhoid surgery. Instruments can be used to either excise or evaporate the tissues. When used as a cutting instrument, the technique is the same as that of scalpel. The duration of wound healing is almost equal to any other techniques. However, there is higher risk of anal canal stenosis.

Recently portable laser equipment are available. Optical fibres directly to haemorrhoidal nodes deliver the laser energy. The laser energy induces destruction of vascular endothelium and thus obliterates the blood flow to the haemorrhoid and so it shrinks in size. The new fibrous tissue formation produces adhesion and thus prevents recurrence.

8.5.2.5. Haemorrhoidectomy by Ultrasonic Scalpel (HUS)

Harmonic scalpel relies on ultrasonic waves producing simultaneously cutting and coagulation effect with minimal lateral damage to the adjacent soft tissues and minimal bleeding. That is why this method is known as Bloodless Ultrasonic Scalpel Haemorrhoidectomy (BUSH). It is indicated in 3rd and 4th degree haemorrhoids

9. STAPLER HAEMORRHOIDOPEXY

The technique is also known as Procedure for Prolapsed Haemorrhoids (PPH). The rationale for stapler haemorrhoidopexy is based on the concept that interruption of superior and middle haemorrhoidal vessels and upward lifting of prolapsed anorectal mucosa and repositioning of the vascular cushion back into the anal canal cause the haemorrhoidal tissue atrophy.

This technique addresses the theoretical concept that the haemorrhoid represents the downward sliding of anal canal lining which results in elongation and kinking of the upper and middle haemorrhoidal vessels. Since there is no disruption of the anoderm, the postoperative pain is markedly low. The anorectal anatomy is restored by returning and fixing the haemorrhoidal cushion to the anal canal. The operating times is shortened, shorter hospital stay, and earlier return to normal activities by the patient are the advantages of this method. Stapled haemorrhoidopexy is safe and effective treatment for large symptomatic haemorrhoids and has fewer early and late complications compared with closed haemorrhoidectomy.

9.1. Operative Technique

A modified 33 mm Circular Stapler is used for stapler haemorrhoidopexy (PPH). The PPH set consisting of a circular stapler, a suture threader, a circular anal dilator, and a purse string suture anoscope. Once the reducibility of the haemorrhoid is established, the anal canal is gently dilated and circular anal dilator is introduced and fixed to the perineum.

The purse string suture anoscope is introduced and a purse string sub mucosal suture, using non-absorbable monofilament suture, is placed approximately 4 cm above the dentate line. Care should be taken to include only the mucosa, sub mucosa, and avoid inclusion of the muscular layer of rectal wall within the purse string. In women, the vaginal wall should not be included. The placement of the suture ' bites' should be close together to ensure that the suture line forms without gab. The open circular stapler is passed through the purse string and the purse string suture as it is tied snugly to the post between the anvil and the shaft and the suture ends are threaded to the shaft with the help of the suture threader. As the stapler is tightened, it is advanced into the anal canal to ensure that the stapler line is several centimetres above the dentate line and it is fired. Wait for a few minutes to give compression over the suture line, and rotation of the instrument should be done to ensure it has cut the mucosa circumferentially and remove the stapler carefully. The suture line is checked for any bleeding and for the suture, line is intact. The mucosal doughnut should be checked for completeness. The circular anal dilator sutures are cut and it is removed.

10. DOPPLER GUIDED HEMORROIDAL ARTERY

LIGATION (DGHAL)
This is the latest, most innovative technology and emerging as minimal invasive procedure of choice in haemorrhoids all over the world. The basis of the technique is restore the haemorrhoids back to their anatomical position and occlude the blood supply to the vascular cushions forming the haemorrhoids resulting in their shrinkage.

AIGNER et al in 2004, reported in their study that the superior rectal artery, compared to healthy volunteers, and the blood flow was really three times higher in patients of symptomatic haemorrhoids. Their study provides strong evidence that the arterial blood flow is related to the development of haemorrhoid cushions. Normally only three arterial branches have been described. However, when detected through Doppler probe, the number may vary from 12 -15. The superior haemorrhoidal artery may not course in exactly defined positions of rectal mucosa (left lateral and right anterior and posterior positions).

10.1. Procedure

In DHAL a specially adapted Proctoscope with an in built Doppler probe which is used to detect feeding haemorrhoidal artery which is subsequently ligated, via Doppler machine with display graph and built-in printer and HAL proctoscope(fig 8.06). A miniature Doppler ultrasound device, inserted into the and canal and rectum, locate branches of arteries supplying the haemorrhoids 2-3 cm above the dentate line by arterial sound of Doppler and also the graphs at the screen. This also provides information of the depth of the artery and facilitates ligation. As soon as the blood vessels are tied off, the Doppler sound disappears and the haemorrhoid shrinks immediately. Usually about 4-5 branches are ligated with 2/0 vicryl on 5/8 the circle needle with taper end. Prolapsing third and 4 th degree haemorrhoids need Recto anal a repair (RAR). This is done with equipment called RAR equipment.

10.2. Recto anal repair.(fig 8.07)

The scope is inserted into the rectum and focused on the site of prolapsing haemorrhoids, first suture is taken deeper to fix tissues, and then the sutures are continued below stopping just above the dentate line (fig 8.08). The last suture is taken after removal of the RAR scope. When the suture is tightened the haemorrhoidal mass is pulled up and ensure its fixation leading to mucopexy (fig 8.09). Thus, almost normal looking anal opening is left at the end of the procedure. Because the sutures are placed in the rectum where virtually no pain sensory nerves the procedure is painless. Sitz bath is not necessary.

The method selected for the treatment of haemorrhoids must suit the need and not the fancy of the patient or the surgeon. Even though one technique is superior to another, any technique that produces a bad result is likely the result of poor judgement or improper execution. Non-surgical treatment is likely to remain the main stay in the management of haemorrhoids. In spite of established standard in different surgical procedures, each case must be judged individually, depending upon the circumstances, be medical, economical, or some special aspect. All will agree that conservative medical, conservative non-surgical, and finally surgical management is the proper route to go in the management of haemorrhoids.

The paradigm shifts, in the treatment of haemorrhoids, is from the concept of haemorrhoidectomy in whatever the form, to the preservation of haemorrhoids while treating the prolapse. The surgical procedure performed should be replacement of the cushions in their normal place and not excision.

11. POST OPERATIVE COMPLICATINS FOLLOWING HEMORRHOIDECTOMY

11.1. Post-operative Pain

Fear of pain is the most important reason why patients avoid surgery in haemorrhoids. The pain may be persistent discomfort and or painful spasm. The persistent discomfort is due to the raw area and lasting for a day or two. The pain due to spasm is caused by the contraction of the anal sphincter. Movements may precipitate these spasms. The most painful period in almost every case is, that is associated with first bowel movement. The pain is managed with analgesics and nonsteroidal anti-inflammatory agents, Sitz bath and laxatives. The pain is markedly less in stapled haemorrhoidopexy and DGHAL.

11.2. Urinary retention, Postoperative bleeding, and wound infection are common in all perianal surgery and are managed accordingly.

11.3. Faecal impaction

Faecal impaction follows incomplete bowel action. Though the bowel opens every day, it is incomplete. Faecal material remains within the rectum and becomes a hard mass. The patient has a continued sensation of rectal fullness. In severe cases, anaesthesia may be required for digital evacuation.

11.4. Anal stenosis (see chapter anal stenosis)
The cause of postoperative anal stricture is excision of considerable portion of the anoderm and anal mucosa. The fibrous tissue proliferation leads to scaring and contraction of the anal orifice and narrowing of anal out let. The stenosis may be within the anal canal or in the anal verge. The stricture is usually short and continued to the mucosa and sub mucosa. In severe cases the lumen may not admits the tip of the finger. If the stenosis is within the reach of the finger regular finger dilatation or with Hegar dilator may provide good results. Severe cases the anal stenosis is corrected by ano plasty.

11.5. Incontinence (see chapter Incontinence)
Anal leak or soiling is common during the early postoperative period but frank incontinence is very rare. After 6-8 weeks, most patients with imperfect continence regain full control. Anal dilatation at the time of haemorrhoid surgery may result in some loss of control of motion or flatus. Loss of anal canal sensation due to removal of sensory bearing anal canal epithelium and replacement with scar tissue may be the cause in some cases. In closed haemorrhoidectomy, this complication never occurs.

11.6. Late complications are anal fistula, skin tag; ectropion and mucosal prolapse are some of the rare complications followings haemorrhoid surgery.

12. HEMORRHOID INSPECIAL SITUATIONS

12.1. Thrombosed external haemorrhoids
Thrombosed external haemorrhoids, is a perianal hematoma present as a painful, pea size, tender mass in the perianal region frequently following an episode of constipation or diarrhoea. The pain reaches the peak in 24-48 hours and start subsiding from 3rd day, the over lying skin

may necrosis and ulcerate leading to bleeding, infection, and discharge. If the patient presents within 48 hours with severe pain, removal of perianal hematoma under local anaesthesia is advised. It there is only discomfort, and 48 hours after the attack, the hematoma is in resolving stage. Conservative treatment in the form of Sitz Bath, stool softener, Bulk forming fibre diet, and analgesics should be advised.

12.2. Thrombosed internal haemorrhoids

This is often attributed to prolapse of the internal component with inadequate reduction resulting is venous stasis and thrombosis of the vascular cushion. Powerful sustained straining at defecation may leads to prolapse and thrombosis of the internal haemorrhoids. The presence of gangrene, prolapse, and oedematous haemorrhoids usually causes severe pain and foul smelling discharge. The treatment of prolapsed haemorrhoids is reduction of the prolapse into the anal canal. Ideally, the patient should be admitted and haemorrhoidectomy should be done on the following day. If the patient had trouble with internal haemorrhoid prior to this episode of thrombosis, advised early surgery.

In the past surgeons were reluctant to do surgery for the ulcerated and gangrenous haemorrhoids for the fear of complications following infection. Now under antibiotic cover it can be operated as an emergency. Emergency surgery for prolapsed haemorrhoids is technically easy and the patient is relieved from pain remarkably.

12.3. Strangulated haemorrhoids

Prolonged swelling of the third and 4th degree haemorrhoids can make it irreducible, leading to incarceration and strangulation. If not treated, may lead to necrosis, gangrene, and ulceration. The patient should be admitted and haemorrhoidectomy preferably, by open technique on the following day should be done.

12.4. Haemorrhoids in pregnancy

During pregnancy, haemorrhoids can occur and it resolves usually after delivery. Conservative treatment is advised. Surgery is indicated only for acute thrombosed prolapsed haemorrhoids. Surgery may be done under local anaesthesia in left lateral position. Sclerotherapy for haemorrhoid in pregnancy is contra indicated.

12.5. Immuno compromised patients

Though Human Immuno compromised Virus (HIV) disease is not absolute contraindication for surgery, these patients should be operated with extreme caution because of high risk of delayed wound healing and septic complications. Surgery is not advised for AIDS patients.

12.6 Coagulation Disorder

All precautions should be taken to prevent bleeding if any surgery is to be under taken.

CHAPTER 6

ANORECTAL SUPPURATION

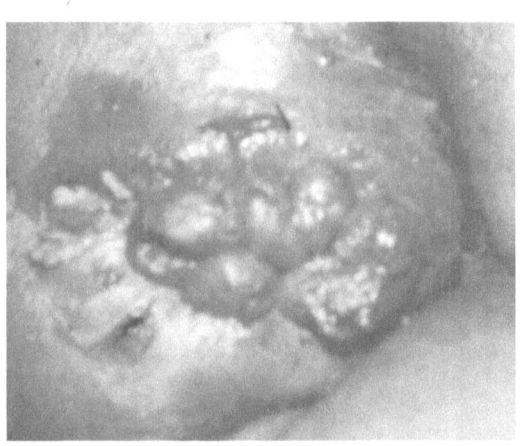

6.01. A case of perianal suppuration

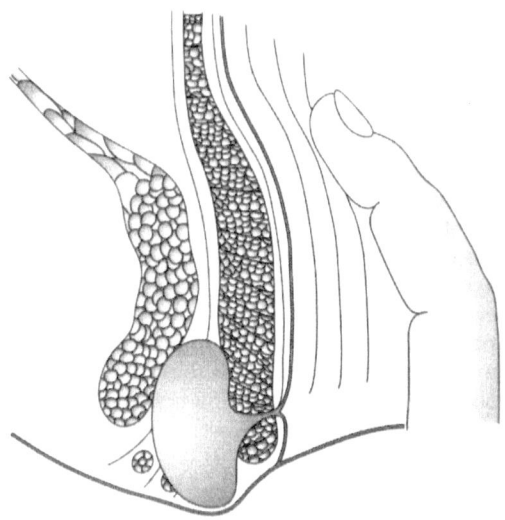

6.02. Perianal abscess- Marginal abscess

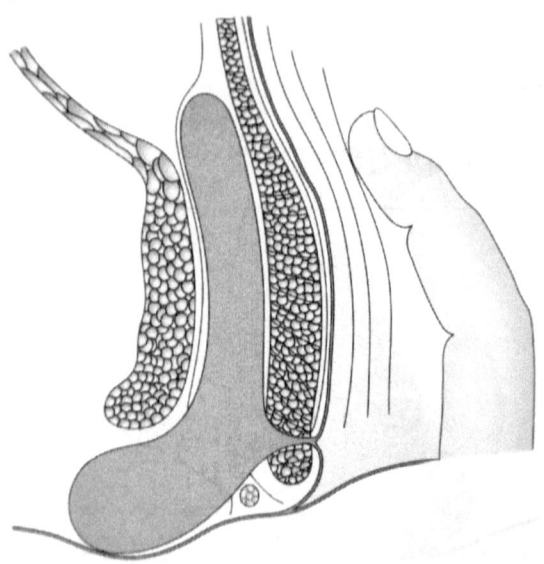

6.03. Inter sphincteric abscess extending above PR sling

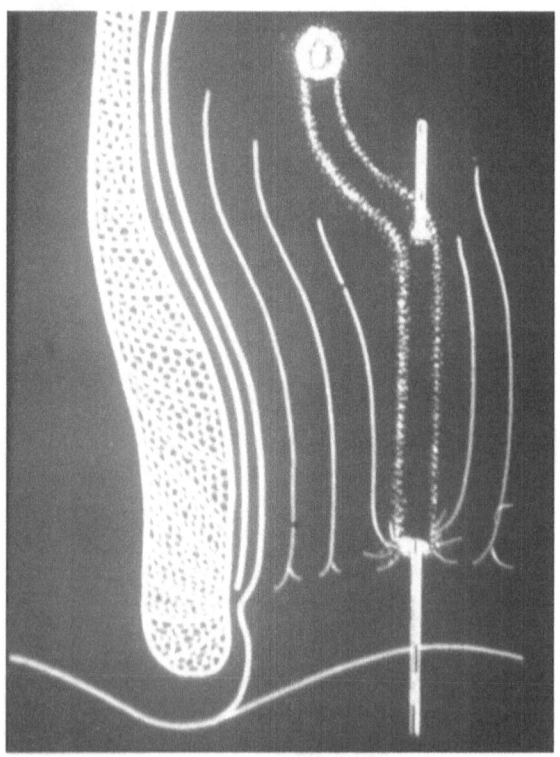

6.04. Sub mucous abscess

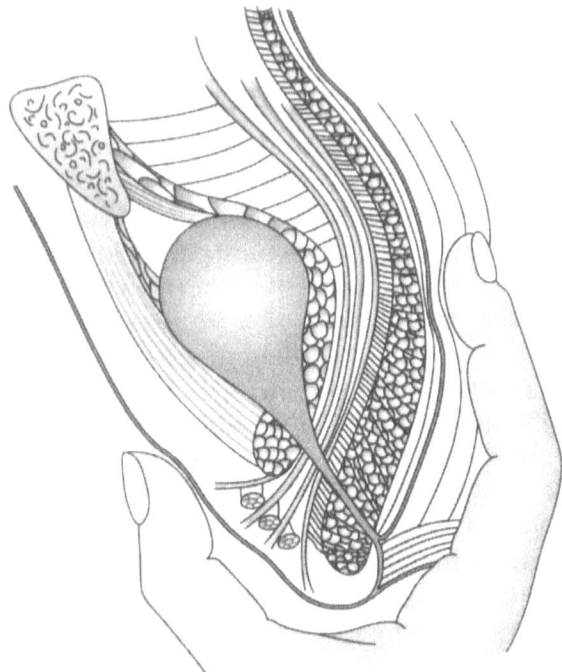

6.05. Deep post anal abscess

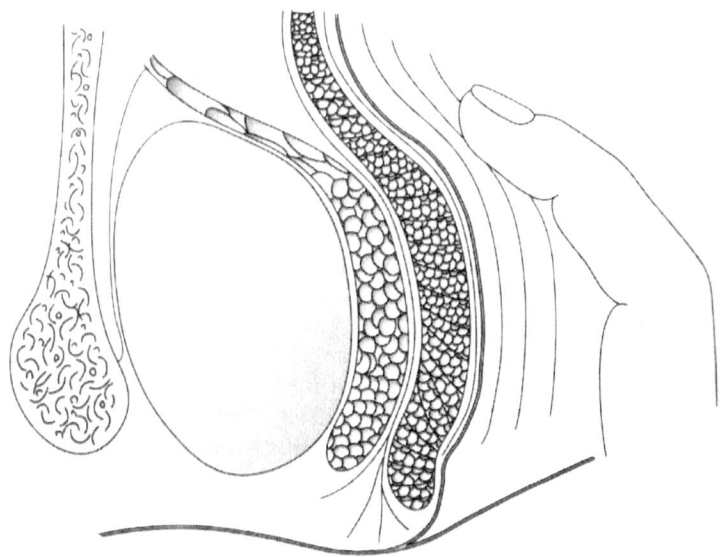

6.06. Ischiorectal abscess

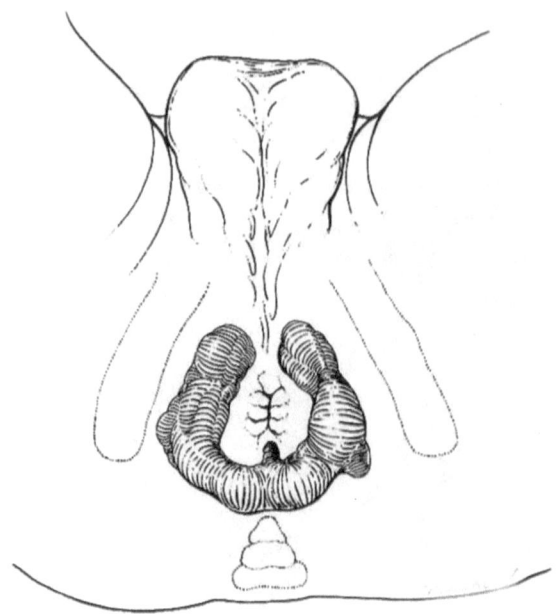

6.07. Horse shoe abscess

Abscess formation around the anal canal and lower rectum is a common condition and has a special importance in relation to anal fistula formation (fig 9.01). Some authors are of opinion that the abscess and fistula, are the same condition and they call them fistulous abscess. However, some cases of perianal suppuration subside with treatment without fistula formation.

1. PATHOGENESIS OF ANO RECTAL ABSCESS

Among various causes of anorectal abscess, the most common cause is Crypto glandular infection.

1.1. Anal glands

There are 8-12 anal glands. The anal glands are racemose type and the gland branches, which end blindly. The duct of this anal gland opens always into the anal crypt. The branches extend over the area for about 1cm enter in to the inter sphincteric area and some of the branches cross the sphincter completely to end in the longitudinal layer. The branches of anal glands do not involve the external sphincter. The anal gland may be infected when the anal gland orifice is obstructed (commonly by the faecal matter) at the anal crypt. In some cases, the anal gland opening may be occluded due to fibrosis of the ductal opening, predisposing for chronic abscess cavity. Whatever may be the cause for the obstruction of the anal grand duct at the anal crypt, a cycle of pathological process occur, duct obstruction- stasis in the gland entry of live bacteria -abscess formation.

The spread of the sepsis is usually caudal, towards the perineum. Less commonly, the sepsis spread upwards resulting in a high intersphinteric or supra levator abscess. Lateral spread passing through the external sphincter resulting in ischiorectal abscess and medial spread the abscess may discharge into the anal canal to resolve spontaneously.

1.2. Causative organisms

Usually it is a mixed infection. The common organisms are Staphylococcus, Streptococcus, E.coli and Proteus. In recent years with regular use of anaerobic culture, it has found out that Bacteriods and clostridium groups of organisms are found to be responsible. Tuberculous infection is responsible in some cases. Severe perianal sepsis with marked tissue destruction may be the presenting symptoms in AIDS.

2. CLINICAL PRESENTATIONS

2.1 Perianal suppuration is more common in male than female and occurs more commonly between 20-45 years of age. It is common in diabetic persons. The representing symptom and severity varies depending upon the type and site of perianal abscess. Anyhow, the pain is the most common presenting symptom. The pain may be in the perianal, perirectal, or deep rectal. It is constant not related to bowel movements, but pain increases on changing the position (sitting and walking). Fever, urinary retention may the associated symptoms and rarely sepsis leading to Fournier's gangrene.

Very rarely the patient may present with no localising symptom or signs of sepsis. Symptoms may be masked in Immuno compromised patients. In AIDS patients sepsis and failure to respond to conventional therapy is a common feature. Metastatic sepsis and severe necrotizing gangrene is now well-recognized complication in AIDS patients with low C D 4 count.

2.2. Because of severe pain, and spasm of the anal sphincter, there may be reflex spasm of the urogenital diaphragm and the patient may develop retention of urine.

3. CLASSIFICATION OF ANORECTAL ABSCESS

The purpose of classification is to alert the surgeon, the likely hood of occult component of the abscess. Even in case where a superficial abscess is visible, one must consider the possibility of deeper collection of pus.

3.1. Perianal (marginal abscess)

The perianal space is a potential space in the area of anal verge. Most anal infections lead to abscess either commence in the intersphincteric space (inter muscular space) or involves it at an earlier stage. The intersphinteric abscess commonly directed downward by the perianal facial septum and present as perianal or marginal abscess (Fig 9.02). The perianal abscess originating from a posterior crypt will tract circumferentially forwards one or other side of the anus to form a large abscess, still confined to perianal space but extending well in front of anterior anal margin. Most of the perianal abscess arises posteriorly. The initial cellulitis may involve a wider area to the sacral tuberosity. Spontaneous resolution of perianal infection is uncommon and it does not improve with antibiotics.The abscess is usually large with thick creamy pus under tension. Untreated, the abscess may discharge spontaneously either into the anal canal or more commonly on to the Perianal skin within 5 cm. Occasionally an area of gangrene may be seen in the skin overlying the abscess when the patient first seen. The pain may of short duration, persistent, troubling, and aggravated, by sitting, walking, and even on coughing

3.2. Inter sphincteric (Inter Muscular) abscess

The abscess, which originates between the internal and external sphincter, passes upwards above the sphincter to form a long finger like projection into the rectal wall (fig 9.03). This type of abscess is also known as Sub mucous abscess(fig 9.04).

3.3. Post anal abscess

The deep post anal space is a potential space lies posterior to the anal canal between the coccygeal attachment of the external sphincter and the levator ani (fig 9.05). Infection in this space can spread on to one or both ischiorectal fossae. The post anal abscess is localized to the posterior aspect of the anus and the anal canal. It may occur with marginal space infection deep to anal fissure. This abscess is related to the anal aspect of internal sphincter.

3.4. Ischiorectal abscess

The ischiorectal space extends up to the sloping roof formed by levator ani muscle, down to the perianal facial septum, which separates it from perianal space. Medially the space is related to the sphincter of the anal canal and laterally it is limited by the facia over the obturator internal muscle. Posteriorly it extends to the sacrotuberous ligament and the lower edge of the gluteus Maximus muscle. The ischiorectal space communicates with each other posteriorly through the deep post anal space (fig 9.06). Most ischiorectal infections seem to originate in the midline in this deep post anal space(fig 9.07). The ischiorectal space is filled with large lobules of fat, which is relatively avascular.

Therefore inflammation is liable to end in necrosis and Suppuration. Untreated abscess rupture throws the perianal skin or into the anal canal. The abscess may penetrate the levator ani muscle, or on rare occasion, the abscess ruptures through the posterior wall of the superficial Perianal pouch and the pus tracts into the scrotum in male or discharge into the vagina in female.

3.5. Pelvirectal abscess

This type of abscess lies above the levator ani muscle has a close relation to the rectal wall. Unlike the Pelvic abscess, it is extra peritoneal. It is a rare condition and not related to anal crypt or anal gland infection and may originate from pelvic pathology such as appendicitis or diverticulitis. In this condition toxic symptoms are marked. Rectal examination may reveal a large, tense, tender swelling outside the rectum palpable well above the anorectal ring.

4. DIAGNOSIS

In great majority of cases of anorectal abscess, the diagnosis is obvious but sometimes the clinical distinction between the different types of abscess is not so easy. Inter sphincteric and perianal infections are more common. Here the pain is the most important symptom. If the intermusclar abscess is situated above the sensitive area of the anus the pain may be less and the patient may complaints of feeling of some heaviness in the anorectal region. There will be an area of cellulitis close to the anal margin with tenderness.

In ischiorectal abscess, the pain may not be severe but the toxic symptoms are marked. There may be slight bulge in the skin over the ischiorectal fossa with evidence of cellulitis. Palpation may reveal tenderness and indurations. Rectal examination will show a large, tense, tender swelling outside the anal canal, which may extend above the level of anorectal ring.

A low inter muscular abscess forms a tender localized lump. The deep post anal abscess may not cause visible swelling but there will be localized tenderness just behind the anal verge at 6 o'clock position, which can be confirmed by rectal examination. In female anteriorly situated abscess may be mistaken for Bartholonian gland infection.

Because of the great distress due to pain and the morbidity involved in delayed diagnosis of anorectal abscess, it is a surgical emergency to decide the line of treatment. The patient may not co-operate for rectal examination. In some cases CT, MRI, or Radio nucleotide white cell scanning may the useful.

5. TREATMENT

5.1. Principles of treatment

i. It is rare for cellulitis around the anal canal to resolve completely without suppuration. Incision should not be delayed with the hope that infection will subside or the belief that pus has not yet formed.
ii. An anorectal abscess appears to have crypto glandular origin. The abscess will tend to recur or a fistula may form and persist until the underlying cause has been removed.
iii. The fistula that follows the surgical treatment of the ano rectal suppuration is due to the presence of the internal opening and not due to the fault in the management of the abscess cavity.
iv. There is very limited place for the antibiotics in anorectal infection for the following reasons. a) Antibiotics do not remove the cause of the infection. b) Pus forms early and antibiotics are not effective in the presence of pus. c) Following the drainage of pus there is rapid recovery and so antibiotics may not be needed after drainage of pus.

However, antibiotics are definitely indicated in a diabetic patients and immuno compromised patients. When the infection is extensive and spreading, antibiotics have a definite place. Anti-biotic may be used during surgical drainage to avoid an episode of septicaemia and they are definitely advised in patients with valvular disease of the heart or those who have prosthetics implants.

5.2. Incision And Drainage

5.2.1. Decompression of Anorectal abscess to allow resolution of acute inflammation and pressure and eventually the pain. If the drainage is done under anaesthesia excision of the crypto glandular origin and the definite fistula procedure may be reasonable. However, there is increased risk of creating false tract and damage to the sphincter mechanism. The incision is made over the maximum swelling or tenderness. The incision must be as close to the anal verge as possible. It will make the fistula tract short if it occurs later.

5.2.2. When the correct site and level is reached, while doing incision, the pus will flow. After the pus is drained, excision of the corners of the wound at least in two places for continuous drainage. Digital breaking of loculations should be done to avoid pocketing of pus. A light packing for 12-24 hours is usually enough to control bleeding if any. Generally packing is removed after 24 hours. After incision and drainage, the inflammation may subside completely. Regular follow up is necessary for the recurrence of abscess or the fistula formation. In a majority of cases, the inflammation subsides to leave a fistula tract, which should be treated as a second stage operation.

5.2.3. One stage operation

The aim of the one stage operation for perianal abscess is drainage of the pus and at the same time preventing the formation of fistula later. This has to be done under anaesthesia either spinal or general. A linear incision is made over the swelling sufficient to admit the finger. When the main gush of pus is coming, specimen taken for bacteriological Examination and culture. The abscess cavities is thoroughly explored with index finger breaking the septa gently and bring the subsidiary abscesses into the main one. Care should be taken to avoid injury to the pudental nerve branches as well as the sphincter. A probe is passed through abscess tract to find out the internal opening and the tract is laid open. The cavity is packed with dry gauze loosely. The dry gauze will not stick to tissue because it will be soaked by the discharge. Petroleum jelly gauze is not advisable.

Disadvantages of one stage operation.

i. It may be difficult to make out the internal opening.
ii. If the internal opening is not made out, the operation is a failure one.

iii. As the tissue is friable during infection false passage may occur.

iv. Long-term follow up shows higher rate recurrence of fistula.

6. HIGH INTERSPHINTERIC (INTER MUSCULAR) ABSCESS

The high intersphinteric abscess needs special attention. Under anaesthesia the offending crypt, is identified by a streak of pus from the anal crypt. It is usually in the mid line posteriorly. A hooked probe is introduced into the opening of the crypt. The abscess is incised and the incision is extended to free the probe. The edge of the incision is to be trimmed. Generally the abscess cavity is drained by opening the inter sphincter space. The whole abscess cavity is opened and curetted. By definition, it is a primary internal fistulotomy in these cases. Repeat examination under anaesthesia may help to ensure adequate drainage.

7. ISCHIORECTAL ABSCESS

Because of the tendency of the ischiorectal abscess to loculate and have high extension, it is often difficult to drain or breakdown the tissues adequately under local, and it is better to drain under regional or general anaesthesia.

7.1. Modified Hanley Procedure

The principle of this technique is decompression and drainage of ischiorectal fossa and deep Post anal space with excision of the primary Crypto glandular origin and placement of drain or Seton to allow resolution of acute inflammation, pressure, and pain.

8. POST ANAL ABSCESS

Isolated post anal abscess is difficult to diagnose. Only under anaesthesia, by digital palpation it may become apparent. The natural extension of post anal abscess is to one or both ischiorectal fossa. The horse shoe abscess is really a Bilateral ischiorectal abscess originate from the deep post anal space infection (fig 9.05). It is preferably to treat post anal abscess with primary fistulotomy and drain through the anal canal. This leaves a portion of external anal sphincter intact and allows the abscess to drain adequately into the distal anal canal. In this way the integrity of distal part of the anal canal and the length of the anal canal are maintained for subsequent healing.

9. POST-OPERATIVE CARE

Once the abscess is adequately drained, the patient is treated symptomatically. Antibiotics may be required in selected cases and diabetic patients and immuno compromised individual. Sitz bath twice a day is advised. The operative wound is checked regular intervals until wound heals by secondary intention. Drainage if kept during surgery has to be removed in 48 hours. Laxative if necessary may be advised for regular bowel action.

CHAPTER 7

FISTULA IN ANO

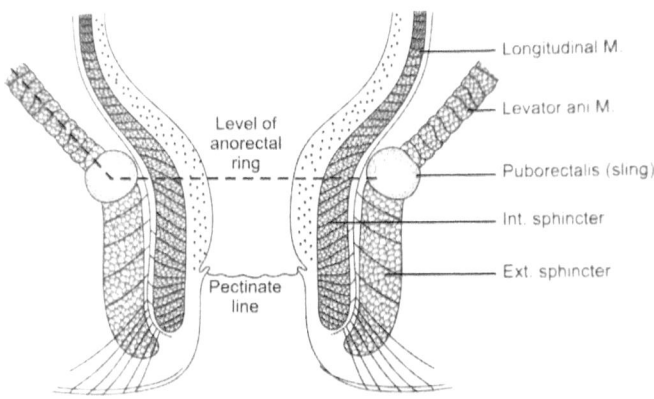

7.01. Anatomy of Anal canal musculatures

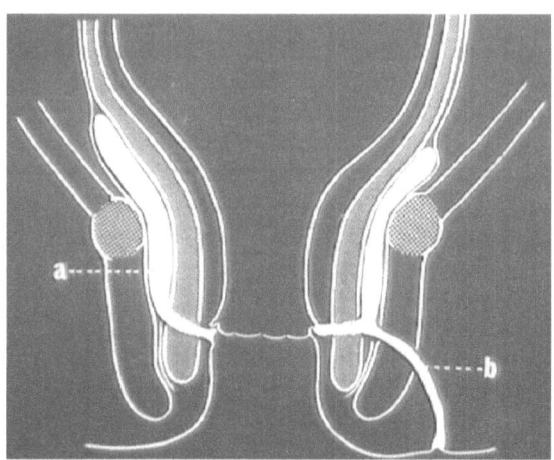

7.02. a) Inter muscular fistula
b). Inter muscular and trans sphincteric tract

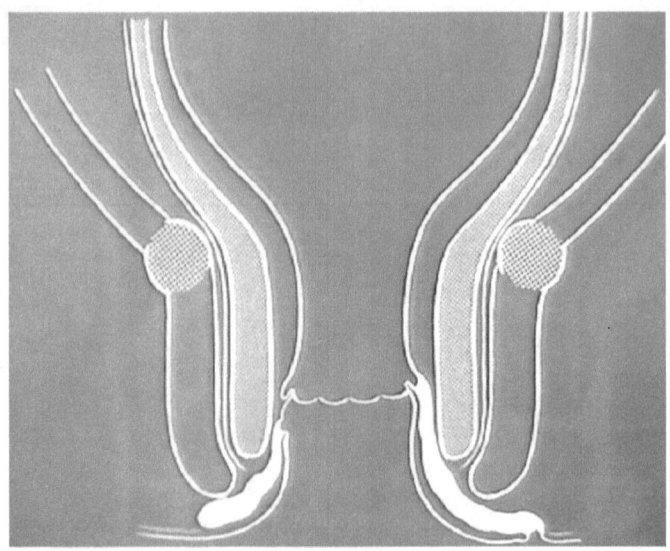

7.03. Subcutaneous fistula

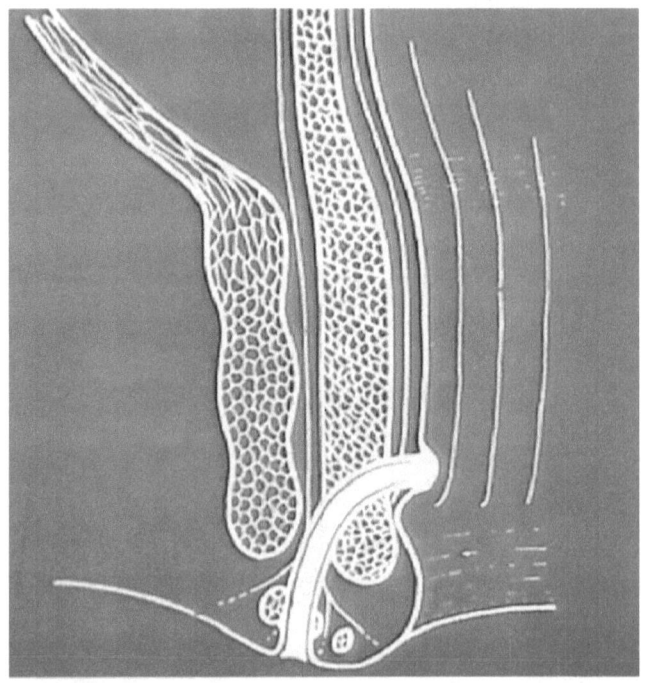

7.04. Low anal fistula

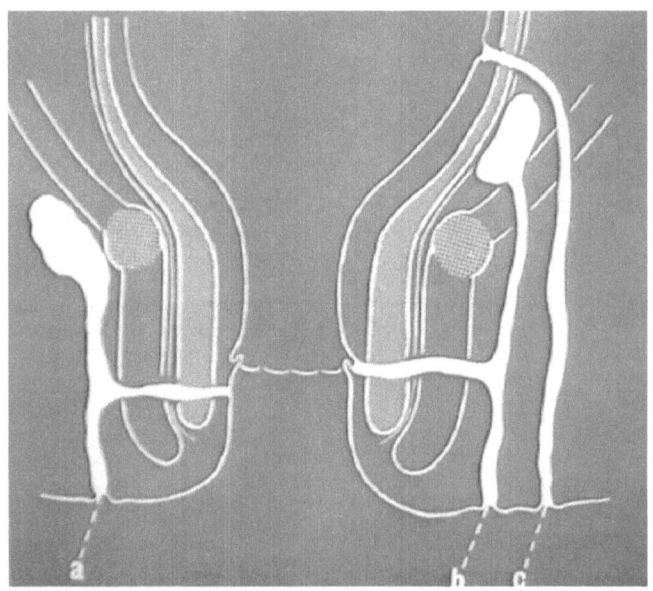

7.05. a) Ischiorectal infra levator tract
b) Ischiorectal supra levator tract
c) Anorectal fistulous tract

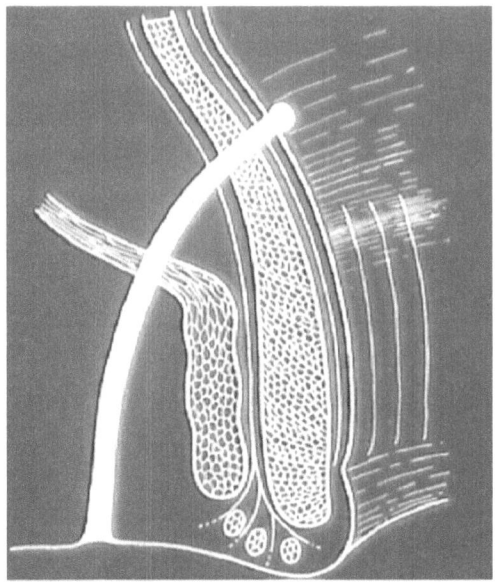

7.06. Anorectal fistula(extra sphincteric)

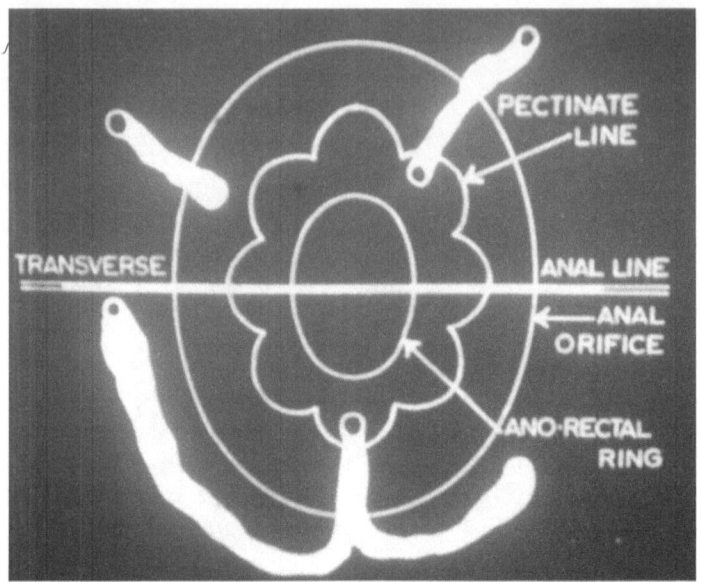

7.07. GoodShalls rule

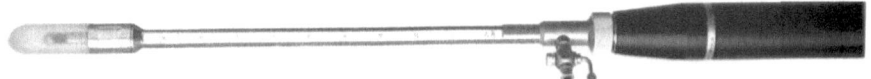

7.08. Endo anal 360 degree rotatable Ultra sonogram probe

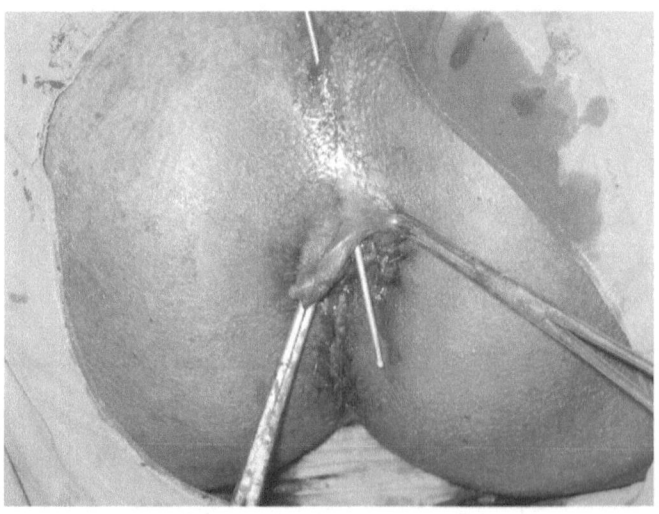

7.09. Probe passed through the tract

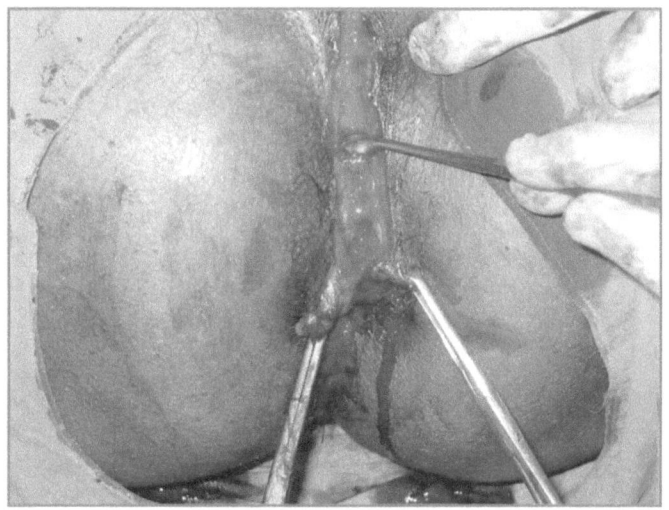

7.10. Curreting the granulation tissue

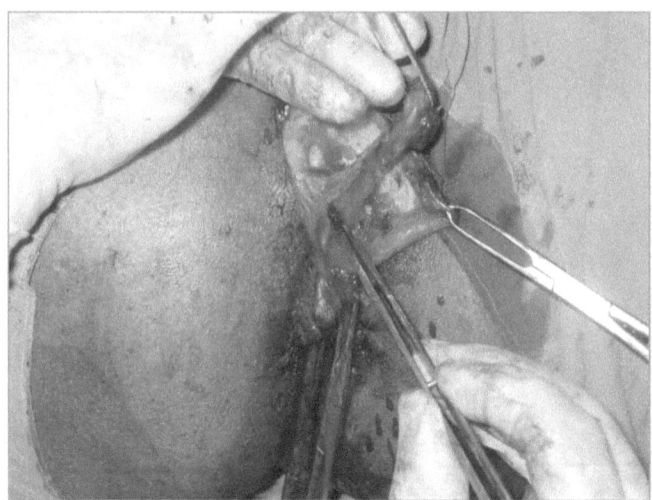

7.11. Excision of the tract

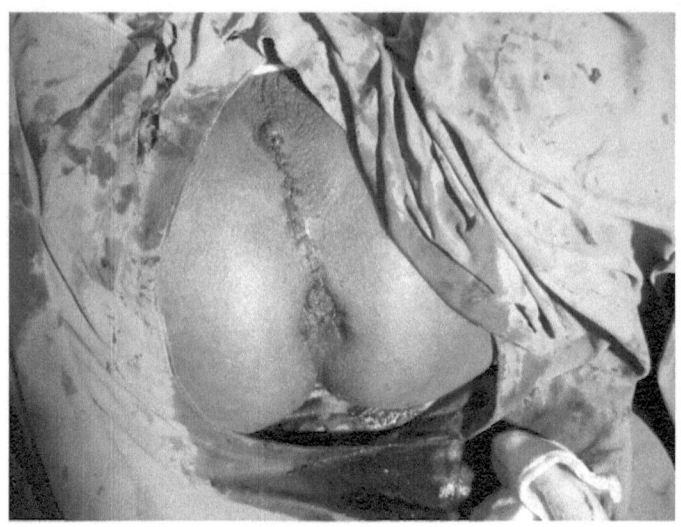

7.12. Fistulectomy with primary closure

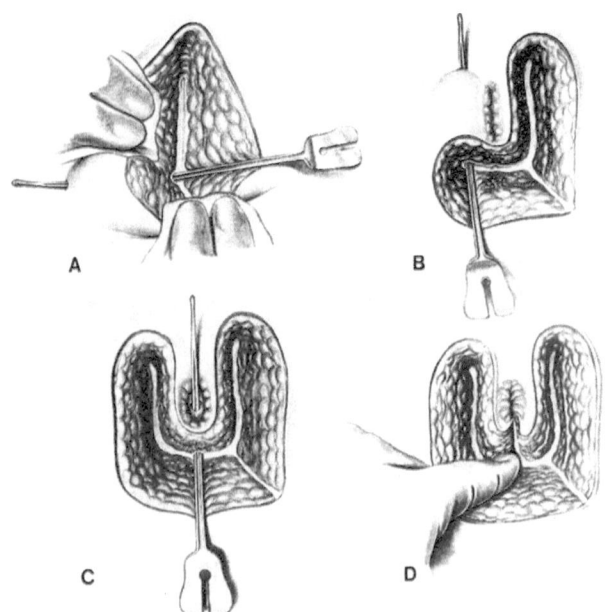

7.13. Horseshoe fistula
c) Showing deep posterior anal tract
d). Deep posterior anal tract laid open

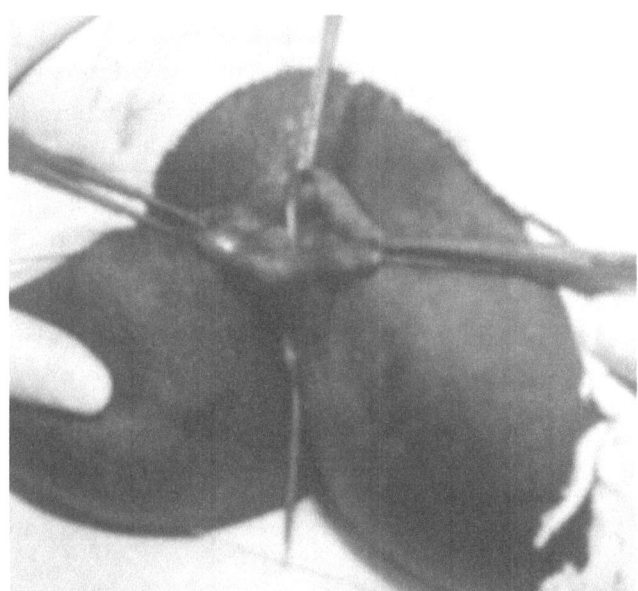

7.14. Subcutaneous tract

Fistula in ano is a tract lined by granulation tissue, which passes, usually from the anal canal to the perianal skin. Medical personnel know anal fistula since antiquity. In Hippocrates period and it was called as Tubercle of Hippocrates. Paulus in 600 A.D. expressed the view that all the anal fistulae could be cured, if both internal and external openings were found. When Felix operated Louis XIV in 1686 for fistula, the anal fistula become the popular disease. According to Park, anal fistula is a granulation tissue lined tract kept open by an infecting source - the anal gland.

1. AETIOLOGY

Fistulas in the vast majority of cases arise from the existing abscess. Eisenhammer is of opinion that the fistula and the abscess are the same condition with the same aetiology. The abscess represents the acute stage of the infection whereas the fistula represents the chronic stage. The infection may be specific or non-specific.

i. Faecal matter obstructs the ducts of anal glands causing stasis, infection and abscess formation. This abscess extends vertically and circumferentially in the plane of least resistant where loose areola tissue and potential space is presents.

ii. The infective organisms are of mixed type both aerobic and anaerobic. The common organisms are Staphylococcus, Streptococcus, and E.coli and Proteus. In recent years with more regular use of anaerobic cultures, it has been found out that Bacteriods and clostridium group of organisms are also responsible.

iii. The specific infection may be due to tuberculosis, Lympho granuloma Venerium.

iv. Fistulous abscess is quite common in Crohn's disease and ulcerative colitis.

2. SURGICAL PATHOLOGY

2.1. Most anal fistulas appear to originate in the crypt of the anal gland or in the anal gland itself. The anal gland, its duct and crypt all constitute the Crypto glandular Complex. The crypto glandular Complex varies in number from 8-12.(fig 10.01). The anal glands branches into a racemose structure, which ends in cystic dilatation. The branches extends over an area of 1cm enter into the internal sphincter and some of the branches cross the sphincter completely to end in the intersphinteric space. The ducts of the anal gland open in the crypt in between the columns of Morgani.

2.2. Infection within this crypto glandular complex leads to an abscess which inturn ruptures usually onto the perianal skin. The corresponding crypt is retracted into a funnel shape by the pull of the fibrous granulation tissue deep into the internal sphincter. It is unusual to see any granulation tissue at the internal orifice. However, the external orifice of the fistula has a characteristics volcanic appearance.

2.3. Most of the external openings are patent with granulation tissue with thin serous or purulent fluid discharge. But in some cases the external opening may close over from time to time. The fistulous tract is lined and filled by unhealthy granulation tissue. The wall of the tract is composed of dense fibrous tissue, which can be felt through the skin by Bidigital examinations. Since maximum number of anal glands are situated in the posterior part of the anal canal, majority of internal opening of the fistula are seen posteriorly.

2.4. Tuberculous fistula. The external opening of the tuberculus fistula are multiple, with ragged, discoloured (blue vice), undermined edges and the tract is not indurated. In these cases signs of active or stigma of previous pulmonary tuberculosis may be detected. The prevalence of tuberculus fistula is probably, underestimated in those places where tuberculosis is common. A routine biopsy should be done is all cases of fistula operated either the excised tract or curetted granulation tissue. With specific anti tuberculus treatment, some fistula may heal without surgery. Persistence and recurrence are common without correct diagnosis and anti-tuberculosis therapy.

3. CLASSIFICATION OF FISTULA

3.1. Park's classification

Park's classification is based on the anatomical basis of the fistula tract in relation to the anal sphincter muscle. Accordingly, the fistula is classified as

i. Inter sphincteric.
ii. Trans sphincteric.
iii. Supra sphincteric.
iv. Extra sphincteric.

3.1.2. Inter sphincteric fistula
In between the internal and external sphincter there is a potential space, known as intersphinteric space, filled with loose areola tissue, lymphatic,

and a few blood vessels. Many of the anal glands components lie in this plane and infection readily travels up and down in the intersphinteric space. All fistulas arise from the infected anal gland, so there is always a potential opening into the anal canal at the dentate line, in some cases this may have been occluded by fibrosis. The fistula tract starts at dentate line and may extend upwards in the intersphinteric space and may reach above the level of the anorectal ring (fig 10.02 a and b). It may present as a Pseudo polypoidal mucosal elevation. The tract could be palpable throughout lengths and for this reason, it is thought that it lies in the sub mucosal plane. Due to downward extension, the intersphinteric tract may open in the perianal region and present as perianal fistula(Fig 10.03).

3.1.3. Trans sphincteric Fistula
The fistula tract passes through both external and internal sphincter and it is related to the upper part of the sphincters but does not extent above the anorectal ring (Fig 10.04.). It may be a true fistula, with an internal opening anywhere from the dentate line to just below the anorectal ring, but usually at the dentate line, or a blind external fistula with the closed end of the tract reaching to the point anywhere up to the anorectal ring but usually with additional blind side tract extending through the external sphincter to the end of the inter sphincteric septum at the level of the anal valve (Fig 10.05).

3.1.4. Supra sphincteric Fistula
The tract extends above the level of the anorectal ring and it lies close to both anal canal and lower part of the rectum. Usually that part of the tract which lies above the ring to be a Cul de sac. However, there may be exceptionally an internal opening in the rectum above the ring. The fistula then either has an external opening alone or more usually there is an internal opening into the anal canal anywhere between the anorectal ring and the anal orifice.

Due to obliquity of the levator ani muscle it is quite possible for a fistulous tract to raise above the level of the anorectal ring and yet be entirely within ischiorectal fossa, separated from the lower rectum and the levator ani muscle and its overlying fascia. This is the common finding in the majority of anorectal fistula and this type is called infra levator anorectal fistula.

3.1.5. Extra sphincteric Fistula

A fistulous tract may pass from an external opening to the rectum above the anorectal ring (fig 10.06). Majority of extra sphincteric fistula are iatrogenic. It may be due to:

i. Difficult Anal surgery.
ii. As a complication of very low restorative resection of rectum.
iii. Result from pelvic abscess.
iv. Gynaecological diseases that have penetrated the pelvic diaphragm and may discharge through the buttock. The tract does pursue an intersphincteric course and the internal opening in the rectum is not necessary in the midlines posteriorly.

4. ISCHIORECTAL FISTULA

In 80% of ischiorectal fistula, the infection originate in the midline posteriorly and 20% in the mid line anteriorly. The posterior ischiorectal fistulous tract is short, which always present, passes directly posteriorly into the deep Perianal space. The internal opening is constantly present either in the dentate line or in just one side immediately below the anorectal ring.

In some cases this posterior fistulous tract is the only tract present which open directly into the skin. The ischiorectal rectal fistulous tract may extend to one fossa only or both and have a horseshoe appearance. The base of the horseshoe lies in the deep Perianal space. The tract lies deeply in the fossa often very close to the rectal wall. Occasionally there is an upward extension through the levator ani muscle.

The external opening is usually 5 cm from the anal margin.

Horseshoe fistula may occur at different levels related to the anus, anal canal, and lower rectum. The position of the actual horseshoe fistula tract is remarkably constant. It hugs the puborectalis muscle and its forms a sling around the sides and back of the anorectal junction, lying external to the upper most part of the external sphincter and below or external to the lower most part of the levator ani muscle. The tract in the ischiorectal fossa passes deep to the inferior haemorrhoidal vessels.

5. CLINICAL PRESENTATION

Anal fistula may result after spontaneous drainage of an abscess in the perianal region or drained by a surgeon. However, in some other cases it seems to occur as relatively minor episode of discomfort associated with some intermittent and sporadic drainage.

5.1. External opening
The external opening of the fistula tract is represented as exuberant granulation tissue. Depending up on the site of the external opening, the type of fistula can be suspected. When the opening is nearer to the anal orifice the fistula is superficial or intersphinteric. If the opening is further away from the anal canal a trans sphincteric component is usually present. When the external opening is near the prominence of buttock, it is often associated with a high fistula, ischiorectal fistula extension, or a supra levator fistula(Fig 10.05). Multiple fistulous openings are usually seen in horseshoe fistula. However, is more common in tuberculosis with characteristic features. Crohn's disease can cause multiple fistulous openings. Sometimes there may not be external opening and the tract may be draining back into the anal canal. Very rarely there may be two different fistulas particularly when there are two or more external openings.

5.2. Internal opening
Irrespective of the number of external openings, the internal opening is single at the level of the dentate line. Presence of a hypertrophied anal

papilla is the direct evidence of the internal opening in the crypt related to that papilla.

In rectal examination, the internal opening can often felt as a dimple or indurated area. The internal sphincter is palpable as an indurated area due to inflammation.

5.3. In some cases the fistulous tract could be palpable in the perianal region, starting from the external opening, towards the anal orifice.

5.4. Goodsalls Rule

Fistulas with their external opening in front of the trans anal line generally has a direct course to the anus, while those with external opening behind this trans anal line take a curved course to reach the anal canal in the midline(Fig 10.07).

One modification was made in this rule, if the anterior external opening is 3 cm away from the anal margin it may have a curved course and opens in the anal canal posteriorly in the midline.

This rule cannot be applicable in multiple fistulous openings, fistula in malignancy and in Crohn's.

6. INVESTIGATIONS

Different diagnostic methods are available for preoperative evaluation of perianal fistula. Accurate preoperative assessment is necessary in all complicated fistula for planning the most suitable surgical procedure.

6.1. Fistulogram

Fistulogram may be useful in recurrent fistula or when high fistula is suspected, or when the external opening is at unusual sites, far away from anal margin like, in the scrotum or gluteal region. Fistulogram does not show the relationship of the tract to the sphincter and so it has a little role in present status.

6.2. Endoanal Ultrasonography (EUS)

It is more useful when residual or secondary tract with abscess is suspected. EUS is a safe and economical technique. EUS is also useful in patients who cannot undergo MRI because of obesity or metallic implants such as pacemakers.

i. EUS is done using a rigid endoanal 10 mh2 rotation Probe. Recently rotating10mhz probe and surrounding cone for 360-degree endoanal ultrasound (fig 10.08) are available. It provides high-resolution images of the anatomy of anal canal including any sphincter defects that may have impact on continence in postoperative period. It is accurate in identification of the course of the primary and secondary tracts

ii. EUS combined with hydrogen peroxide (HPUS) as a contrast. Hydrogen peroxide as a contrast media improves visualizations and provides an accurate preoperative assessment of the fistula. When hydrogen peroxide is introduced through the external opening, a fistulous tract appears as hyper echogenic. The external opening must be visible to introduce hydrogen peroxide, which is a limitation for HPUS.

iii. The use of 3 D images provides more information on the anatomy of the anorectal disorders.

6.3. Magnetic Resonance Imaging (MRI)

MRI provides excellent image of the anatomy of the pelvic musculature and the surrounding tissues. There are number of studies demonstrating the occurrence of fistula or abscess, seen in MRI. are compared with operative findings. Now MRI is regarded as the investigation of choice to define the anorectal sepsis and fistula. Contrast MRI show the tract and abscess around the fistulous tract much clearly than ultra sonography. Like EUS the pathology in ischiorectal fossa and the evaluation of the supra and infra levator extension could not be made out. MRI does not accurately distinguish the internal sphincter and mucosa.

6.4. Anorectal Manometry

Anal manometry provides informations of internal and external anal sphincter functions. Voluntary contraction during Manometry will provide a reasonable assessment of puborectalis and external sphincter activities. Manometry study of the maximal resting pressure and squeeze pressure may be useful guide to predict which patient may go for incontinence and may be useful in deciding the type of surgery for the particular case.

6.5. Fistuloscopy

More recently, Anorectal fistuloscopy by using flexible ureteroscope is one more armamentarium for the Anorectal surgeon. Intra operatively, the internal opening, multiple complex tracts, and iatrogenic tracts can be easily identified. In some centres, this technique is used to curate the granulation tissues of the tract.

The choice of technique of various investigations, like any other modern investigation, depend on expertise and availability of imaging technique in the centre.

7. TREATMENT

The surgical treatment is always a balance of curetting the inflammatory process and preservation of sphincter functions. It is wise to remember the warning given by Lockhart Mummary that '' failures are common and more reputations are lost in the treatment than with any other operations". Few problems in surgery need much more judgment as the treatment of complex fistula. The consequence of injudicious therapy with recurrence and incontinence may be disasters. JC. Goligher stated that at least half of the patients seen by him with fistula have already had one operation for this condition.

7.1. The basic principles of fistula surgery

i. Identify the internal opening.
ii. Identify the course of the tract.

iii. Ensure drainage of both internal opening site and the tract.

iv. Attentive postoperative care.

v. Follow up to ensure proper wound healing.

7.2. Once the fistula becomes apparent, it rarely heals. The fistula is kept open by the infected anal gland and if it is removed, the fistula will heal. On Bidigital rectal examination, if the tract is felt, it is passing superficially. If the tract is not felt, it will be heading upwards to the roof of the ischiorectal fossa from external opening, before turning an acute angle to open into the anal canal at dentate line.

7.3. Two important parameters determine whether the fistula can be laid open, or treated by staged procedures.

i. The relationship between the internal opening and anorectal junction

ii. A patient with bowel movements of 3-4 times /day with low Resting Pressure will have a high chances of faecal soiling or even incontinence.

8. FISTULECTOMY OR FISTULOTOMY

Fistulotomy is lay open the tract for every superficial fistula with minimal resulting damage to the sphincter muscles. In Fistulectomy, the fibrous tract is excised taking care not to damage to the sphincter.

Under anaesthesia, a probe is passed through the external opening, taking care to avoid creating a new tract by forceful advancement. If the probe cannot be passed through the external opening, a partial external fistulotomy may help to pass the probe. If the probe successfully passed through the tract into the internal opening, a careful assessment of the sphincter left below the tract and the tract is laid open, the granulation tissue is curetted and sent for the Histopathological examination. If excision of the tract is planned, the tract is completely excised up to the internal opening and excision of part the mucosa over the internal opening for removal of infected anal gland and proper drainage at internal opening operative steps shown in(figs10.09, 10.10, 10.11, 10.12).

8.1. Marsuplization after fistulotomy, that is suturing the skin edges to the fistulous tract to accelerate the healing, can be done in selected cases.

8.2. Some surgeons advice excision of the fistulous tract for the following reasons. i. Prevention of recurrence of the fistula from the residual anal gland. ii. The wound healing occurs quicker. iii. When the tract is left, rarely cancer may from the residual epithelium.

8.3. Most fistulas are perianal or low intersphinteric and the tract passes through the lower part of the internal and external sphincter (Fig 10.11 a and b). As a rule, division of the sphincters below the fistula tract does not disturb the function, provided the puborectalis muscle is not damaged.

8.4. Fistulectomy with primary sphincter reconstruction. After the fistula tract is excised the divided anal sphincter is reconstructed. The success rate is high and the and the postoperative continence power is good and incontinence is avoided. Anal manometry results were improved in many cases when incontinence was present pre operatively.

8.5. Minimal excision of skin edges facilitates quicker healing and less scar tissues, and more supple perianal skin when healing is complete. When the wound is wider, then suturing of the wound either partially or completely has to be done.

8.6. Place of Seton. Complex fistula and high Trans sphincteric fistula are managed in stages and application of Seton. Monofilament non-absorbable suture material is used in Seton. The fistulous tract is land open, curetted and excised close to the lateral wall of the rectum or anal canal, the internal opening and the surrounding mucosa and sub mucosal layer is excised trans analy. The inter sphincteric tract is curetted for granulation tissue and a non-absorbable monofilament suture is passed through the intersphinteric tract and tied loosely. It will allow continuous decompression of the tract, and allow the tract to collapse. Seton is applied for those cases where there is increased risk of incontinence, particularly in elderly patients and those with chronic diarrhoea. Extra sphincteric fistula associated with trans sphincteric component in the anal canal needs to be treated appropriately or simultaneously.

A loosely tied Seton can act as a drain, promote fibrosis, and as a marker in staged Fistulectomy. In cutting Seton the monofilament suture is tied tightly, and this cutting Seton slowly divide the internal anal sphincter. By dividing this sphincter slowly, retraction of the ends of the divided sphincter muscle is prevented.

9. HORSESHOE FISTULA

It is a bilateral ischiorectal fistula with a post anal component (fig 10.13 a and b,). The entire horseshoe fistula tracts are unroofed. The fistulous tract is opened from its external opening in a horseshoe fashion and the post anal fistula component is opened into the anal canal(Fig 10.14).

10. LIGATION OF INTER SPHINCTERIC FISTULOUS TRACT (LIFT)

This procedure consists of ligation and division of intersphinteric fistulous tract in the intersphincteric space and curettage of the remaining tract. The postoperative pain is less and the wound heals much faster.

11. VIDEO ASSISTED ANAL FISTULA TREATMENT(VAAFT)

A recent technique for the treatment of anal fistula. The operation is performed by a 18 cm long rigid fistula scope with 8° angled eye piece. The fistula scope is passed through the external opening to the level of the internal opening. The lining of fistula tract is cauterized by unipolar electrode, Endobrush is used to brush out the cauterized fistulous lining, and necrotic materials are evacuated by washout. The internal opening is closed by either mucosal flab or by stapler. The technique, efficacy, and recurrence of fistula are being studied in different centres and awaiting for the final report.

12. DIODE LASER

This is a recent technology. Laser energy is delivered by optical fibre, into the fistulous tract. The laser energy causes destruction of fistula epithelium and the fistula tract is obliterated by shrinkage.

13. FIBRIN GLUE

Autologous fibrin glue is used in complex anal fistula. The technique involves curettage of granulation tissue in the tract followed by injection of autologous fibrinogen, and thrombin. Thrombin activates the fibrinogen and the resultant formation of Fibrin, plugs the fistula tract. This is contra indicated in the presence of sepsis.

14. ANAL FISTULA PLUG

The commercially available Biological Fistula Plug is inserted into the internal opening of the fistula and fixed in place with one or two stitches for fixation of the plug for preventing migration. The external opening is enlarged or excised in a limited area and a fistula probe is passed to the level of the internal opening. If the internal opening is retracted, limited mobilization of mucosal edge is done. The collagen plug is kept in antibiotics solution for 2 minutes for hydration. The hydrated plug is passed through the internal opening to the tract and is pulled out to the external opening. The plug is pulled through the external opening till the plug sits snugly. The excess plug at external opening is trimmed at external opening. Anal fistula plug is used in Crohn's fistula, and patients with poor anal sphincter function. This technique needs further studies for the long-term results.

15. POLYMETHYL METHYL-ACRYLATE CO-POLYMER (PMMA)

After partial excision of the tract 1-3 chains of 10-30 small beads (each 4-5 mm in diameter) of PolyMethyl Methyl Acrylate co-polymer (PMMA) were inserted. Each beads contains 7.5 mg of gentamycin sulphate, and 20mg of zirconium dioxide (contrast media).The gentamycin prevents sepsis and recurrence.

16. AYURVEDIC THREAD

A technique first described 3000 years ago by SUSHRUTA for the treatment of fistula using medical Ayurvedic thread as a temporary drainage seton. Studies are on progress to compare the continence and recurrence rate of Ayurvedic thread treatment of fistula with fistula surgery.

17. POST-OPERATIVE CARE

Unless contra indicated, the patient is allowed normal diet from the first post-operative day. There is nothing is gained by delaying the first bowel action. Once the motion is passed, a light protective dressing is advised. Adequate attention to the wound healing during postoperative period is necessary. Neglect of this aspect of treatment may easily result in recurrence of fistula in spite of well-performed operation. The aim is sound healing by granulation from the depth of the wound and prevention of premature contact between the opposing skin edges and granulating walls.

17.1. The wound should be reviewed periodically. If at any stage, there is dissatisfaction with the course of healing, the patient must be re-examined in the operation theatre and the edges of the wound should the separated. Care should be taken that, the wound fills up from bottom outwards, because the edges may unite without obliteration of the dead space leading to recurrence.

17.2. Silicon sponge may the used to prevent premature closure of the wound. It can be done by the patients themselves.

Daily sitz bath at least twice a day is advised till the wound heals. It promotes wound healing by increasing blood supply by vasodilatation and the discharge of the wound is washed out.

19. RECURRENCE

Even in experts hands recurrence after fistula surgery occurs, only the percentage of recurrence that counts. In fact, if anybody says that there is no recurrence of fistula after fistula surgery done by him means that he openly accepts that he has not followed the cases properly.

19.1. A fistula wound never heals and the recurrence of the fistula may present from the time of surgery. It may be due to the infective source is not removed completely. Alternatively, a recurrence may not be apparent for many years. Some patients develop a new fistula altogether.

19.2. A recurrent fistula should arouse suspicions of Crohn's or tuberculosis or any other specific cause for the fistula, which may needs elaborate investigations.

19.3. It is important that before surgery, the patient should make to understand the necessity for careful postoperative regime. It is unwise to attempt an accurate pre-operative forecast of the definite period of covalence after a fistula surgery.

19.4. It must be admitted that fistula operations have an inevitable reputation for subsequent recurrence is not infrequent and impairment of anal continence is another unfortunate sequence sometimes encountered. There are few operations in surgery where the quality of the result is so much influenced by the technical skill of the surgeon.

CHAPTER 8

PRURITUS ANI

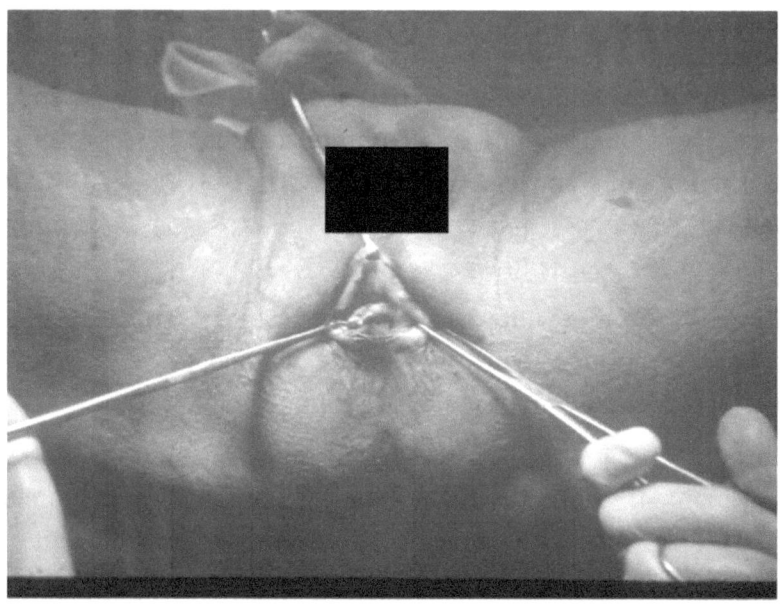

8.01. Hypertrophied anal papilla

Pruritus ani is a symptom complex caused by multiple Pathological states alone or in combinations. This further potentiate 'itch scratch cycle', which often triggers an irresistible urge to scratch and can lead to perianal excoriation to frank ulceration. Significant number of patients has pruritus caused by extremes of hygiene. It is the commonest complaint in colorectal practice and occurs more commonly in men. The rich nerve supply to the perianal region is thought to be the primary cause for the sensitivity to potential irritation.

1. CLASIFICATION

i. Primary (Idiopathic).

ii. Secondary.

1.1 Primary Pruritus

The primary pruritus is not associated with detectable underlying disease and the aetiology is normally obscure. It is suggested that it is an allergic phenomenon due to sensitivity to some items of the diet or other allergic agents.

1.2. Some suggest that the pruritus is due to irritation of the perianal skin by faecal contamination even when there is no gross soiling is evidence. Poor anal hygiene is a common cause. Obese persons with funnel shaped anus and elderly debilitated persons have difficulty in mechanical cleanings. In same way, diarrhoea and anal incontinence may predispose for pruritus.

1.3. Coffee is the most common cause of primary pruritus. The other foods which produce pruritus are Tea, Chocolate, excessive dairy products, spicy foods, citrus fruits and tomatoes.

1.4. Lanolin which is the constituents of many skin lotions. Lotions of many skin medications, used for treating the skin lesions, including topical steroids and local anaesthetic ointment like lignocaine may induce pruritus.

1.5. Psychological background. Stress and mental tension may precipitate pruritus. It is reasonable to assume that severe perianal itching for 24 hours a day, and every day is likely to make an individual rather psychics.

1.6. The anus is one of the erotic areas in the body and the patient have a habit of enjoying the itching with its resulting scratching pleasure sensation.

2. SECONDARY PRURITUS

2.1. Local anorectal lesions

Local anal lesions which cause excessive moisture in the anus, the lesions themselves do not cause pruritus, but secondarily by production of discharge with subsequent irritation and possibly secondary infection may cause the pruritus ani(fig 11.01).The common lesions are fistula, fissures, hypertrophied anal papilla, partial mucosal prolapse of rectum, prolapsing haemorrhoids, large skin tag.

2.2. Faecal contamination of perineum

Poor hygiene is the common cause. Obese persons and elderly debilitated persons have difficulty in mechanical cleaning of the perineum. In same way, diarrhoea and anal incontinence may predispose for pruritus.

2.3. The skin surface in the perineum is covered with a protective film of fatty acid triacylglycerols, wax esters, which are produced by sebaceous glands and the epidermis directly. These protect the skin from irritation and excoriation. Soap defats the skin and remove this protective substance. Any soapy film that has not completely cleaned from the perineum may cause initiation of the 'itch scratch' cycle.

2.4. Thread worm infestation

It is the common cause of pruritus in children. The main complaint is a crawling sensation in the anus and perianal region than itching and irritation.

2.5. Fungal infection

The common type of fungal infection is Candida Albicans which is saprophytic yeast found in the face and the skin. Invasion of skin by the yeast may occur when the anoderm is damaged by trauma, and use age of steroids in heavy doses or heavy doses of antibiotics. Candida infection is common in uncontrolled diabetes. It is suggested, that Candida is often a secondary invader on any moist excoriated skin. Female patients may have existing genital yeast infection in leucorrhoea. Candida Albicans are equally distributed in the perineum with or without pruritus.

2.6. Anal Papilloma

Papilloma arising from anal skin is caused by Human Papilloma Virus. These lesions are also called anal warts and condyloma acuminata. They are common in young men with homosexuality.

2.7. Systemic diseases
Uncontrolled diabetes, Leukaemia, Lymphoma, Jaundice, and Renal failure.

2.8. Systemic drugs
Many oral medications change the faecal pH to alkaline, which exacerbate the symptoms of pruritus. Antibiotic and mineral oil can initiate pruritus ani.

3. PATHOLOGY

3.1. Acute Pruritus
The anus is surrounded by red, oedematous, dry or weeping areas. The whole part of the perianal skin is involved and the vagina in female and in male posterior aspect of the scrotum is involved in some cases.

3.2. Chronic Pruritus
The skin changes involve a smaller area, which may be patchy or diffuse thickened oedematous radiating skin folds from the anus. In advanced long-standing cases, the perianal skin appearance may be those of leukoplakia elsewhere and the changes may extend to the dentate line.

3.3. Microscopic appearance
The epidermis is thickened due to proliferation of the prickle cells hyperkeratosis. The Rete pegs are elongated. The dermis shows generalised mild infiltration of inflammatory cells. There is oedema of the dermis and dilation of the superficial blood vessels and lymphatic and atrophy of the sebaceous glands.

3.4. Once the skin has been broken by scratching, the bacteria gain easy access into the epidermis and dermis and leads to infection.

3.5. Exaggerated rectoanal inhibitor reflex

There is raise in intra rectal pressure during rectal distension and the internal anal sphincter relaxation is greater and prolonged. On this basis of this finding, it is postulated that there is an exaggerated recto anal inhibitor reflex in primary pruritus ani, which results in increased leakage of faecal fluid through the anal canal, accounting for the irritation in pruritus ani. In some cases, the leakage may be secondary to co-existing anal pathology, probably as the result of increased mucous production or by interfering with anal canal closure.

4. CLINICAL PRESENTATION

Itching with varying degrees of intensity in the perianal region and it is more in the night and sometimes it affects the sleep. The symptoms are more in the summer probably due to greater amount of sweating leading to anal moisture. The itching in most cases are with remission and relapsing. Superficial scratch marking and inflammations of the skin can be made out. In chronic cases there is thickened skin with exaggerated and oedematous skin folds.

5. CLINICAL ASSESSMENT

The clinical assessment of patients with pruritus ani must include a careful history to assess the duration of symptoms and severity. History of any potential predisposing pathology like diabetes, gynaecological disorder or inflammatory bowel disease should be elucidated. A psychiatric history and a brief assessment of personality should be done.

Clinical examination includes careful inspection of the perianal region for superficial scratch marks, and presences of faecal matters in the perianal area. Carefully look for the presence of condylomata, skin tag, and other anal lesions. Proctoscopic and Sigmoidoscopic examination should be done. A small portable ultraviolet light can be used to find out the presence of C. Minutissimum.

Anal scraping examination for Mycelia using small scalpel, stool culture for enteric pathogens, stool examination for ova and cyst and parasites. Serological test for syphilis and HIV to be done.

6. TREATMENT

6.1. As majority of cases of pruritus are idiopathic, the treatment is unsatisfactory and the prognosis should always be rather guarded. It is wise to tell the patient that the complaint tends behave in a remissions and relapsing manner.

6.2. Majority of patients believe that either the cancer is responsible for the itch or that cancer will develop if itching is not controlled. A complete anorectal examination including Sigmoidoscopy should be done. After completion to these exhausted examinations, the patient is informed that there is no question of cancer. It is useless and unfair to give such a assurance without complete Anorectal examinations.

6.3 All previously used creams and ointments must be discontinued. Proper anal hygiene should be maintained.

Many patients perceive their problem is due to lack of cleanliness. The opposite is also more likely. Vigorous scrapping of the perianal region with soap and water will cause the skin damage and contact dermatitis may supervene. It is difficult to convince the patient that anal area need not be sterilized. Avoid soap for Perianal cleaning and Perianal wash with water is advised. Avoid alcohol wipes and deodorants in the perineum.

6.4. Diet regulations. Diet regulation may be helpful in certain cases. Restrict flatus forming foods, spicy food, dairy products, Chocolate, and other foods which aggravates the symptoms. Alcohol and coffee should be avoided. Change in the pH of the food and faces may improve the condition. Alkaline powder ingestion increases the pH and Lactobacillus acidophilus decreases the ph. High fibre diet and taking sufficient fluid allow passages of soft motion.

6.5. Some patients may need admission for frequent application of various cooling lotions, and creams. Admissions of the patient enable a fairly heavy sedation, which may inhibit the tendency to scratch and thus interrupt the 'itch scratch' cycle. Zinc oxide cream is use full in the treatment of pruritus ani. It promotes healing process and act like a protective barrier against drainage.

6.6. Potassium Permanganate sitz bath (the water is minimally stained and not in purple colour). Hydrocortisone cream 1-2% applied 2-3 times a day is effective against itching. If there is fungal infection 2%, Ketoconazole cream along with hydrocortisone cream is applied for 3 weeks. When there is bacterial infection and extreme excoriation is present tropical ointment like Polysprin is advised for 10 days.

7. TREATMENT OF ASSOCIATED LESIONS

Thread worm infestation is diagnosed by obviously seeing the worms or demonstration of ova from a strip of cello tape placed in the anal region in the morning before defecation or bath. Threadworm infestation is treated by mebendazole 100 mg tablet and repeated after one week to prevent reinfection. Scabies and Pediculus Pubis are treated by Benzyl Benzoate lotion. It should be applied to the whole body. Pediculus Pubis is treated by Lindane. It is effective in single application. To be repeated after seven days to kill lies emerging from any eggs that might have been survived the first application.

8. SURGERY

Surgery is needed only for the elimination of the underlying pathology for the pruritus. Biopsy is advised when any pruritus lesion does resolve with standard treatment. Obvious lesions like, Haemorrhoids, fissure, fistulas, mucosal prolapse are surgically treated. If a skin lesion prevents adequate cleaning, excision of the lesion is indicated.

For idiopathic pruritus, injection of 20cc of solution containing 15cc of 1% Lignocaine, 5cc of I % methylene blue, and 100mg of hydrocortisone, to the perianal skin under general anaesthesia is advised. It may have to be repeated in some cases.

CHEPTER 9

COMPLICATIONS OF ANAL SURGERY

A complete knowledge of postoperative complications of anal surgery is the first line towards the prevention of complications. Familiarity of the anatomy of the anorectal region and carful techniques are essential for gratifying results. The method selected for the management of anorectal lesions must suit the need, and not the fancy of the patient or the surgeon.

1. URINARY RETENTION

The urinary retention after anorectal surgery is the most frequently seen complication and the incidence varies from 10-30%. It results in discomfort and leads to urinary tract infection.

1.1. Causes of urinary retention in anorectal surgery
i.   Reflex Urethral spasm.
ii. Inhibition of detrusor muscle as the result of reflex involving afferent fibres of pudendal nerve, sacral spinal cord and efferent pelvic sympathetic nerves.
iii. Spinal anaesthesia.
iv. Fluid over loading
v.   Rectal packing
vi. Rectal spasm
vii. Enlarged Prostate in old peoples.

1.2. Management of Urinary retention

1.2.1. It is important to keep in mind that a single episode of over distension of the urinary bladder can produce irreversible damage to the detrusor muscle. So intermittent catherisation with sterile safety precautions when necessary is accepted.

Provide privacy for the patient for micturition. Patient may be asked to site in the in bed or stand by the side of the bed and try to pass urine. If is patient can walk, or permitted to walk in the ward in the first postoperative day and can go to the toilet with one attendee waiting outside the toilet room.

1.2.2. Hot water bag may be applied in the supra pubic region. Injection of carbacol may help to relieve the retention.

2. POST OPERATIVE BLEEDING

2.1. Early bleeding
Early bleeding is due to reactionary haemorrhage from the skin wound or from the pedicle. Massive bleeding in the immediate postoperative period result from loose ligation of pedicle or slippage of the knot. In such case, the patient should be taken to operation theatre and under anaesthesia, the bleeding pedicle is identified and ligated. If there is no obvious bleeding point then the pedicle is over sewn.

2.2. Delayed bleeding
Delayed major secondary bleeding seen most often, after haemorrhoidectomy on the 7th to 10th Postoperative day. The cause of delayed bleeding is secondary to breakdown of granulation tissues during defecation or due to infection disrupting the blood vessels at the pedicle. Secondary haemorrhage is more serious as the bleeding may be considerable and the blood may accumulate in the rectum and escape detection for some time. Inspection of the perineum may show the tickling of dark blood from the anus.

Rectal examination may reveal large soft blood clot and on withdrawal of finger, blood will come out. During proctoscopy, the blood clot may extrude through the lumen of the proctoscope.

2.2.1. Management
Delayed bleeding is usually not a preventable condition. The patient is admitted and vital signs are recorded. Depending upon the general condition intra venous drip is started and fluid replacement should be carried out. If there is marked blood loss or haemoglobin is low, blood transfusion to be given. If there is no improvement in vital signs the patient is examined under anaesthesia, in the operation theatre, the bleeding point is looked for and if could be made out the bleeder is under run using 3/0 vicryl in a small half circle needle. Antibiotics may be necessary in some cases.

3. POST OPERATIVE PAIN

The fear of pain is the most important reason for the patient to avoid surgery in the Perianal region. Moderate pain is unavoidable after anorectal surgery. To reduce the post-operative pain a number of modification of technique of surgery (ex. Closed haemorrhoidectomy) or addition of some technique (ex. anal dilatation, or lateral sphincterotomy) while doing haemorrhoidectomy or using stapler.

The pain is of two types i. Persistent discomfort ii. Pain due to spasm. The persistent discomfort is due to raw area and the incisional wound, and may be there for one or two days and again when passing motion in the post-operative period usually for one or two days.

Spasm pain is caused by the sphincter contraction, which is involuntary. The most painful period in almost every case is that associated with the first bowel action in the postoperative period.

The pain is controlled by frequent administration of narcotic analgesic either by injection or orally. Diazepam for 24 - 4 8 hours small doses are helpful in the decreasing anxiety and muscle spasms.

4. INFECTION

In spite of the presence of large number of Gram negative and anaerobic bacteria in the anal canal, infection after surgical procedures in anorectal region is very low. Still perianal and ischiorectal abscess have been reported. Delayed diagnosis of perianal sepsis leads to disastrous consequences. Any patient with pain and fever and urinary retention after anorectal surgery should be carefully examined for the site of sepsis. When the infection site is identified, the treatment consists of drainage, debridement of necrotic tissue and parenteral antibiotics. For perianal abscess early diagnosis and adequate drainage are essential for successful out come

5. FAECAL IMPACTION

The factors contributing for constipation after anorectal surgery are:

i. Effect of anaesthetic agents.
ii. Post-operative analgesic medications.
iii. Dehydration.
iv. Fear of painful defecation by the patients and so try to avoid.

Faecal impaction follows incomplete bowel action, though the bowel opens every day, it is incomplete and the faecal material remain within the rectum becomes a large hard mass. The patient will have a continued sensation of rectal fullness and leads to faecal impaction and spurious diarrhoea. The diagnosis of faecal impaction in the postoperative period is based on a high index of suspicion and digital examination.

When the diagnosis of faecal impaction is made gentle tap water enema is the first line of treatment. When the enema is not successful, disimpaction of the faecal mass from the anorectum is done by gentle digital examination and the enema is repeated. Some patients may need anaesthesia for digital evacuation of hard faecal mass, flowed by enema.

6. ANAL INCONTINENCE

Varying degrees of mucus discharge, incontinence for gas and rectal soiling are not infrequent after anorectal surgery. After 6- 8 weeks most patients with imperfect continence remain in full control. In general anal continence after Anorectal surgery, in majority of the cases are mild and transit.

6.1. Causes

The anal incontinence after anorectal surgery may be due to i. loss of anal canal sensation due to removal of the sensory bearing anal canal epithelium and replacement by scar tissue. ii. Damage to the sphincter muscle. iii. Creation of Anatomical defect such as keyhole deformity.

Surgery for fistulas is frequently followed by severe anal incontinence. Prevention of this complication may be challenging when operating complex anorectal fistula. As a rule, anal continence is maintained if the anorectal sensory mechanism is preserved and the anorectal angle (Puborectalis sling) is intact.

Exception to this rule occurs, depending on pre-operative functional status of sphincter mechanism.

6.2. The following principles are useful in preventing severe anal incontinence in anorectal surgery.

i. The surgeon must be familiar with the anatomy of the anal, sphincter muscle, and the relation of fistulous tract with the sphincter.

ii. Thorough evaluations of the functional status of the sphincter mechanism by careful physical examination and manometry study, if necessary, before surgery.

iii. In general the entire internal sphincter muscle and much of the external sphincter may be divided in the posterior aspect as long as the Puborectalis muscle is preserved.

iv. Division of the muscle anteriorly should be as conservative as possible because there is no Puborectalis muscle anteriorly.

v. When the fistula tract involves a larger portion of the sphincter, a seton should be applied.

7. ANAL STENOSIS

The cause of postoperative anal stenosis is excision or destruction of considerable portion of anal mucosa and anoderm. Fibrous tissue then proliferates leading to contraction of the skin and narrowing of the anal canal.

7.1. The stenosis may be in the anal verge or may be within the anal canal. The stenosis in anal verge is due to excessive removal of the skin below the dentate line. With each bowel action, the skin splits and a chronic fibrous tissue is formed. The anal orifice is scared and contracted.

The stenosis within the anal canal is due to generous inclusion of anal canal mucosa during surgery. The stricture is short and involves the mucosa and sub mucosa. In severe cases, the lumen may not even admit the tip of the little finger.

7.2. Treatment

7.2.1. Non operative treatment

Mild anal stenosis frequently respond to bulky and stool lubricating agents. Moderate type of stenosis within the reach of finger can be treated with finger dilatation or by Hagar dilator.

7.3.2. Operative treatment

The aim of treatment is to relieve the stenosis without incontinence. The factors influence the choice of operation includes the severity of the stenosis, its location and the cause of the stricture. For anal verge cutaneous stricture, the best approach is to perform four quadrant incisions thorough the scar, followed by dilatation by Hegar dilator. Anoplasty is advised when the defect of the anoderm is extensive. The basic feature of anoplasty for anal stenosis include division of the scar tissue, advancement of perianal skin into the anal canal to increase its circumference.

8. UNHEALING WOUND

The perianal and anal canal wound heal within 2 weeks, because of good blood supply. Even left open, the wounds heal within 8 weeks. If the wound does heal within 8 weeks, exclude Crohn's disease and malignancy. After excluding these conditions Curettage of granulation tissue or copper sulphate application may be useful. If the conservative treatment fails surgery in the form of wound excision and advancement skin flaps are indicated.

9. MUCOSAL ECTROPION (WET ANAL SYNDROME)

The mucosa of the rectum protrude through the anal margin circumferentially is called mucosal ectropion. This is due to advancing the rectal mucosa and suturing to anoderm or anal skin during the performance of anorectal surgery. This deformity results in wet anus (due to seepage of motion) and consequently perianal irritation (pruritus), bleeding, pain, and occasional tenesmus (wet anal syndrome).

Surgery is the treatment of choice, if the symptoms are annoying the patient. The surgical treatment consists of excision of the ectropion, mobilizations of the perianal skin and suturing the mobilized skin with proximal anal canal. The goal of surgical treatment is to restore the ectropion mucosa with the original level proximal to the dentate line.

CHAPTER 10

ANAL STENOSIS

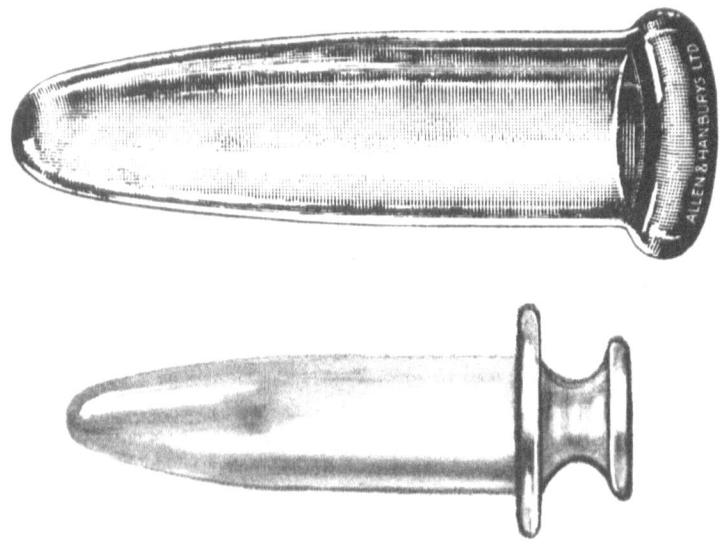

10.01. Anal dilator

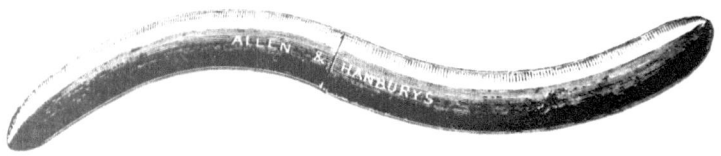

10.02 Hegar dilator

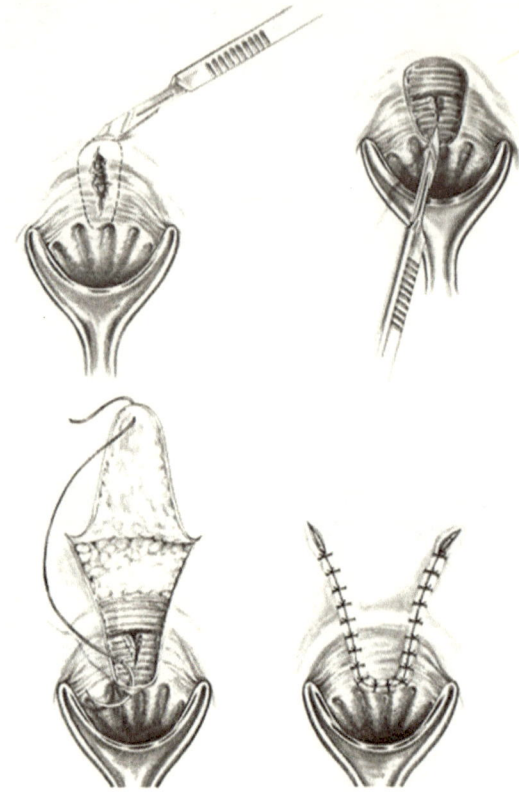

10.03. Local flap

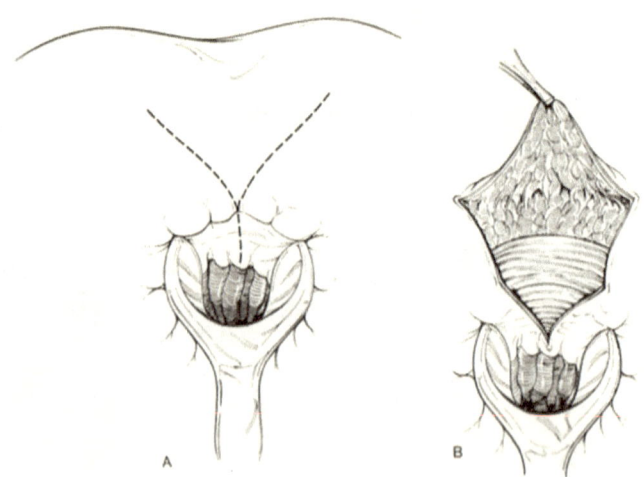

10. 04. Y-V plasty

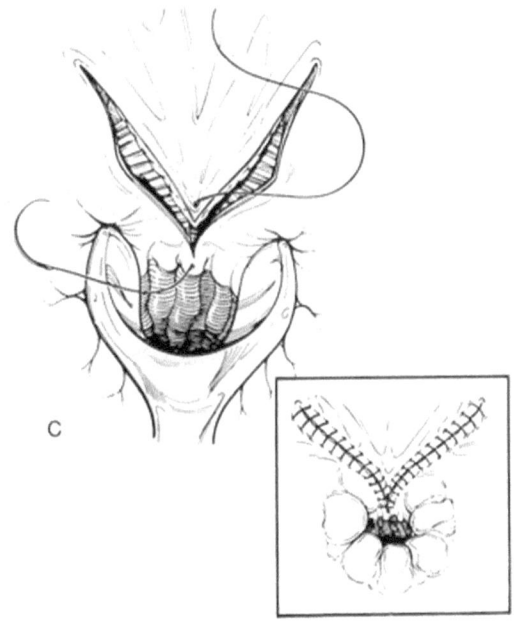

10.05. Y-V plasty

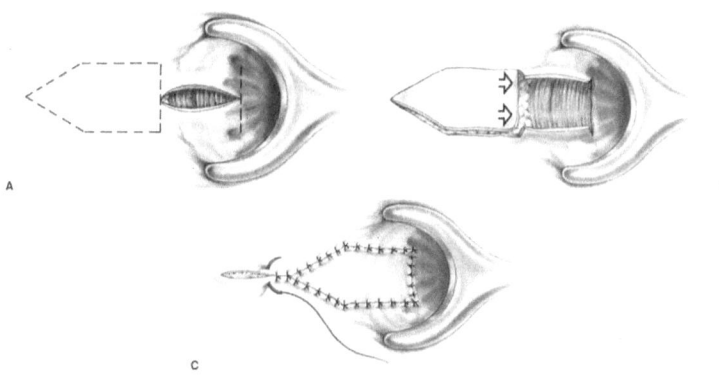

10.06. House flap

Anal stenosis is a condition in which there is mechanical narrowing of the anal orifice and anal canal. There is loss of compliance of natural elasticity of the anal canal opening which ultimately becomes fibrosed and abnormally tight. The anal stenosis may follow any circumstances that cause scaring of the anodermal area.

1. CAUSES

i. Congenital anal stenosis

ii. Iatrogenic. Repeated trauma to anal orifice due to self-habitual behaviour of introducing foreign body into the rectum (auto eroticism) which results in repeated trauma and ulceration of the anal orifice leading to stenosis

iii. Post-operative. Post haemorrhoidectomy stenosis is the most common cause for the anal stenosis. Excessive removed of anoderm during surgery leads to progressive healing by fibrous scar tissues, which may proliferate and contract the anal outlet. The surgeon must always aware of the need to preserve the anoderm when operating in anal canal. Ultra-low anterior resection of the rectum may result in postoperative anal stenosis.

iv. Anal lesions. Paget's disease of anal canal, Bowen's disease of anal canal, anal canal malignancy, and AIDS.

2. CLASSIFICATION

Anal stenosis is classified deepening upon the pathology, level of lesions, and severity of the stenosis.

2.1. Pathological classification

i. congenital. Imperforate anus, anal atresia.

ii. Primary. Involution stenosis in old age

iii. Secondary. Following Surgery in the anal canal, like haemorrhoidectomy.

2.2. Involvement of segment of anal canal

i. Low. Stenosis is at the distal anal canal 0.5cm below the dentate line.

ii. Middle. When the stenosis is within 0.5 cm from the dentate line.

iii. Proximal. When the stenosis is 0.5cm above dentate line.

2.3. Severity of the Stenosis

iv. Mild. The anal orifice admits index finger with some difficulty.

v. Moderate. Need forceful digital dilatation before introducing the index finger.

vi. Severe. Unable to pass the finger even with forceful dilatation.

3. CLINICAL PRESENTATION

There may be no correlation between the clinical findings and symptomatology. Elderly patients may lead a comfortable life in spite of narrow anal canal.

The common presenting symptoms are

i. Progressive constipation, feeling of some obstruction, at the level of anal orifice during defecation.

ii. Pain and bleeding during defecation, when there is a tear, in the anal verge.

iii. Constipation may be so severe that the patient may need digital evacuation leading to further trauma to the anal orifice.

iv. Faecal impaction and overflow incontinence. v. Diarrhoea due to prolonged use of laxatives (Paraffin anus).

v. On long standing cases, there is retrograde distension of the rectal ampulla and the rectum resulting in Mega rectum.

4. PHYSICAL EXAMINATION

Physical examination may reveal the probable cause of stenosis.

4.1. It may be impossible to perform digital examination or the anal orifice may admit only small finger for examination Sometimes it is difficult to differentiate from sphincter spasm associated with anal fissure. Local anaesthetic jelly applied to the fissure with the finger of which the anal orifice admits and waiting from a few minutes abolishes the spasm associated with an anal fissure.

4.2. Presence of scar indicates the postoperative stricture from previous anal surgery.

4.3. In congenital anal stenosis, a ring like narrowing occur in the upper end of anal canal 1 cm from the surface perineum of the new-born, and about 2cm, in old children. Its extent varies from a string like stenosis in a normal anal canal to a diffuse fibrosis involving the internal sphincter. The external appearance is normal and hence the lesion may pass unnoticed for some time. When the child starts taking solid food, the constipation becomes progressive and severe. By the time, the rectum would have gone for considerable secondary dilatation and rectal inertia.

4.4. Patients with long-term laxatives, there is sphincter wasting resulting in anal stricture, a consequence of passing small, narrow faeces over many years. This is probably because of the lubricated stool fails to dilate the anal canal.

4.5. In sodamy individuals, perianal sexually transmitted diseases to be suspected and relevant investigations has to be done.

4.6. Ulcers in perianal region

i. Ulcers with classical clinical presentation of rodent ulcer or squamous cell carcinoma can be easily differentiated and diagnosed.
ii. Paget's disease may be suspected when there is ulcerative, crusty or papillary lesion.
iii. Bowen's disease can be suspected when there is a raised, irregular, scaly, brownish plaque with eczematous lesion.

5. TREATMENT

Medical treatment any alter the defecation but do not treat the cause of the problem namely narrowing of the anal canal.

Surgical Treatment

5.1. Congenital anal stenosis is treated by division of fibrous track by internal proctotomy followed by persistent dilatation. Management may be very tedious, because the external appearance of the anal orifice appears normal in babies, months or even years may pass before the lesion is discovered or significantly appreciated. It is important that the stenosis must be corrected before the child develop mega rectum. The out flow incontinence may be misdiagnosed as due to sphincter inadequacy.

5.2. Excision of the scar tissue and sphincterotomy
The classical treatment for anal stenosis is lysis of the stricture and excision of the scar tissue and the rectal mucosa is sutured to the underlying internal sphincter transversely may give a good result. This is an accepted technique for the mild form and sufficient skin bridge remains. For more profound stenosis, a formal anoplasty should be performed to treat the basic problem of loss of anal canal tissues.

5.3. Mild Stenosis
It can be conservatively managed with fibre supplementation and stool softener. Dilatation of the stenotic area is an important aspect in the management and it is best accomplished by regular passage of faeces, which provide the most natural stretching possible. The patient is advised to have daily dilation at home either digitally or with any mechanical dilator available in the market(fig 13.01, 13. 02). The patient is instructed to sit down as he or she sits for defecation, bear down and gradually insert the dilator. Dilatation under anaesthesia may be avoided as it may cause hematoma formation and further fibrous which may worsen the stenosis.

5.4. Moderate Stenosis
If conservative management in the form of bulk laxative and finger dilatation fails, surgery is needed. In moderate stenosis partial lateral sphincterotomy by open method is advised in which the scared anoderm is also divided. Surgery will relieve the pain and the apprehension that accompanying the defecation.

High fiber diet should be followed. When greater area needs to be covered sufficient skin can be obtained by performing bilateral advancement in the right and left lateral area. This will permit resurfacing up to 50 per cent of anal canal. Postoperative usage of stimulant laxatives or lubricant laxative such as, mineral oil may lead to the danger of narrowing of anus out let to return to previous stage.

5.5. Severe stenosis

In severe anal stenosis there is marked scaring in the anoderm. A number of surgical procedures have been adopted for the correction of severe anal stenosis. Basically all the techniques for treating this condition, are mobilization of anoderm into the anal canal. Replacement of non-pliable tissues with elastic and pliable neo rectum or anal canal is the basis for the surgical therapy of anal stenosis. Advancement flab, transfer, or rotation flaps, are the main technique adopted for corrections. The vascular supply for these flaps is from unnamed vessels that perforate sub mucosal or sub dermal vascular plexus or in subcutaneous tissues. More complex rotation flaps are based upon named vascular pedicles.

The rotation flap can cover a grater surface area without tension than an advanced flap technique. If multiple procedures have already carried out wider area of coverage is needed so rotation flaps are indicated. However, these complex procedures should be done in specialized centres where speciality services are available. Mucosal advancement flap and tissue transfer are more commonly advocated.

5.6. ANOPLASTY (fig 13.03)

Anoplasty is indicated in those persons who had anal stenosis following haemorrhoidectomy, excision of anal canal lesions, and mucosal ectropion. Post haemorrhoidectomy stenosis is usually in the lower anal canal and the cicatrix scar involves anoderm. Occasionally the stenosis may be higher in the anal canal so that the narrowing is actually above the dentate line and partially involves the mucosal aspect of the anus. In these conditions, sphincterotomy along with excision of the actual stenotic ring is advised.

5.7. Y.V. ANOPLASTY

Commonly performed surgery for anal stenosis. It has little morbidly and an excellent functional results (fig13.04, 05). The incision is made radially at the level of the stricture, which forms the vertical line of Y. The wide portion of V is located further out in the perianal area. For proper mobilization, sub dermal dissection is done. The resultant V flap is advanced at the base of the vertical line. Suture dehiscence, ischemic contracture, hematoma, Flap necrosis and stricture are some of the complications following this surgery.

5.8. V. Y. Advancement anoplasty (Rosan)

After excision of the stenosed segment of the anus a V Shaped flap, at least 2 cm length is advanced to the muco- cutaneous junction.

5.9. Mucosal Advancement Anoplasty

An incision is made perpendicular to the dentate line extending into the anal verge. The mucosa is undermined for 2-5 cm. Now the wound will look like a transverse wound. The scar tissue is excised, mucus membrane is excised and the edges of the mucosa are sutured to the distal border of the internal sphincter at the anal verge. The external part of the wound is left open.

5.10. House Advancement Flap (fig 13.06)

The word house demotes the schematic representation of a house in terms of the way the flap is created. The theoretical advantages are that it provides a broader skin flap for the entire length of the anal canal and allows primary closure of the donor site.

5.11. Anal stenosis in Crohn's disease

Anal stenosis in Crohn's disease is not the condition to be treated by any surgical techniques involving extensive undermining or development of flap. It is to be treated by dilatation of symptomatic stenosis under anaesthesia.

CHAPTER 11

FAECAL INCONTINENCE

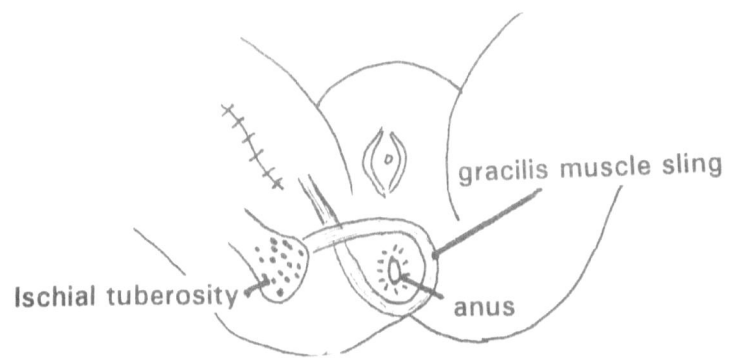

11.01. Gracilis transposition

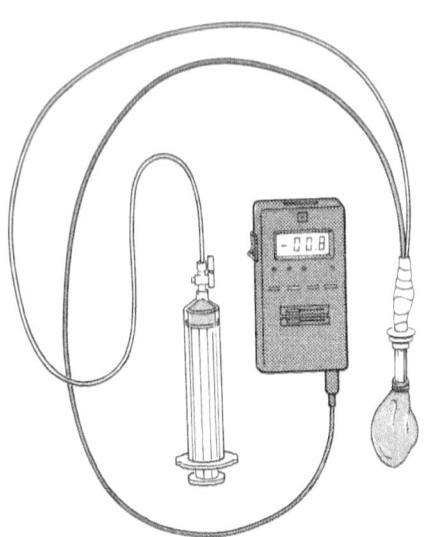

11.02. Bio feedback apparatus. The inflation of balloon is followed by pelvic floor contraction and increased EMG activities

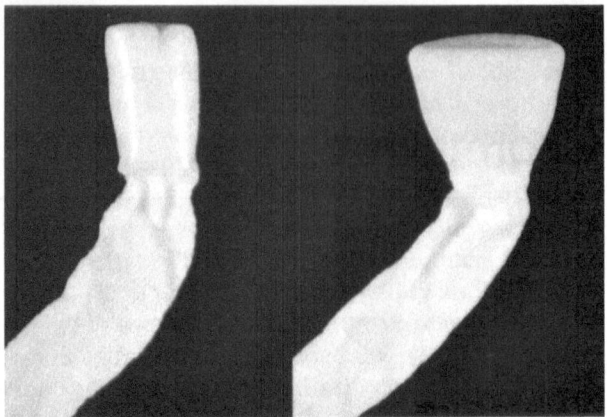

11.03. Anal plug

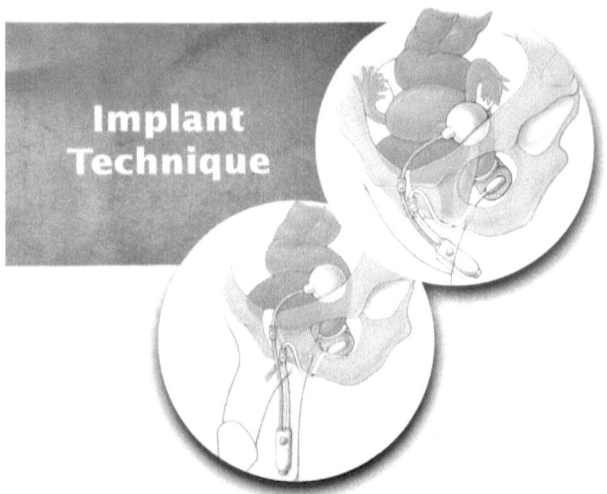

11.04. Implantable artificial anal sphincter

Faecal incontinence is an embarrassing symptom most commonly affects elderly particularly female population. Voluntary control of defecation is essential for normal social wellbeing. Anorectal continence depends on the balance between two aspects, stool consistency and sphincter efficiency. Fine coordination of the internal sphincter relaxation and external sphincter contraction is likely to be maintaining normal continence.

1. ANAL CONTINENCE DEPENDS ON THE FOLLOWING FACTORS

i. Internal anal sphincter.

ii. Pelvic floor function.

iii. Rectal compliance.

iv. Rectal capacity.

v. Rectal sensation.

vi. Colonic transit.

vii. Stool consistency.

viii. Central nervous system function.

2. CLASSIFICATION OF THE INCONTINENCE:

i. True incontinence. Passing faeces without patient's knowledge or voluntary contraction or both.

ii. Partial incontinence. Passing flatus or mucus under the above circumstances.

iii. Over flow incontinence. Result of rectal distension with relaxation of anal sphincters (e.g. Faecal impaction)

3. BASIC ASPECTS OF ANAL SPHINCTER COMPLEX

i. The internal anal sphincter (IAS) is continuation of smooth muscle of the rectum and it is under the control of the autonomic nervous system. IAS is always in tonic contraction and is responsible for 80% of resting pressure.

ii. The external sphincter (EAS) is a striated muscle, which is under voluntary control. It is innervated by pudendal nerve. It remains partially contracted at rest. It contributes 20% of resting pressure of the anus. Inhibition of EAS during defecation allows the passage of stool.

iii. Puborectalis muscle (PRM). It is a U shaped sling around the anorectal junction with 90 ° angle, which closes the pelvic outlet and prevents the passage of stool in normal condition. It remains partially contracted at rest.

Continence is maintained by interaction of a number of factors. The consistency of the faeces, coordinated action of smooth (IAS) and striated muscle (EAS), Puborectalis sling and Pelvic floor musculature and the integrity of autonomous and somatic innervations.

4. ETHIOPATHOLOGY OF INCONTINENCE

4.1. Idiopathic (neurogenic) faecal incontinence

It is defined as progressive loss of anal sphincter function without a history of anorectal surgery, trauma. A gradual deterioration of continence occurs. Neurological diseases like cerebral degeneration, motor neuron disease may affect the bowel control. The common condition that produces neuropathy is diabetes mellitus. The patients are troubled because of diarrhoea from autonomic neuropathy and the sphincter impairment. In neuropathic disorder, the patient is unaware that he or she has passed faeces or mucus. The commonest cause of the incontinence is senile dementia where urinary incontinence also occurs.

4.2. Injury

Injury to anal sphincter mechanism due to trauma or surgery in the anorectal region may result a situation where the patient is unable to prevent the passage of flatus or faeces. Complete incontinence occurs in:

i. Rectal injury.
ii. Obstetric injury.
iii. Following fistula surgery.
iv. Sphincter preserving rectal excision.
v. Prolonged labour.

4.3. Liquid faeces

Incontinence may present in spite of normal anorectal sphincter function, in the presence of large quantity of liquid faeces, conditions like inflammatory bowel disease, irritable bowel syndrome, and gastroenteritis.

4.4. Impairment of rectal sensation

Impairment of rectal sensation can occurs in mesenteric nerve degeneration and from long standing use of laxative, anti-cholinergic or phenothiazine. Overflow incontinence from faecal impaction is common in elderly. Faecal impaction may be caused by neglecting the call to stool, faulty dietary habit, or impaired intestinal peristalsis (delayed colonic transit) difficulty evacuation of hard stool. The so-called incontinence in faecal impaction is spurious diarrhoea, also known as overflow incontinence.

4.5. Sphincter derangement

Internal sphincter is responsible for the greater part of resting tone of the anal canal and continence of mucus and flatus. Continence is maintained by partly under voluntary control by striated muscle external sphincter and levator ani muscle. Partial incontinence occurs following internal sphincterotomy or anal dilatation. Even when the external sphincter is divided, completely satisfactory continence is provided by intact Puborectalis muscle.

When both external sphincter and Puborectalis muscle are divided the patient will be incontinent.

4.6. Sphincter infiltration of anorectal malignancy can cause spurious diarrhoea.

4.7. In most female patients the cause of faecal incontinence is due to, prolonged labour and vaginal delivery, due to damage to pudendal nerve. Anterior sphincter disruption occurs in second stage labour. The sphincter muscle is damaged because of their close association with Perianal body which may be stretched or torn doing vaginal delivery.

4.8. Lower motor neuron diseases

Damage to the somatic afferent and efferent fibres between the anorectum and spinal cord may occur in lesions of lumbosacral spine such as cauada equina, spondylosis, tumours, and secondary to intra pelvic lesions involving the sacral plexus.

4.9. Encopresis

Encopresis or psychogenic soiling is defined as passage of formed or semi-solid stool in children under cloths, that occurs regularly after the age of four years. It is essentially an involuntary evacuation of the bowel not caused by organic factors. It is more common in male children and is analogous to enuresis.

5. CLINICAL EXAMINATIONS

The single and most important feature in clinical evaluation of anorectal incontinence is, it affects on social activities and work life. A detailed history of continence is important in determining the severity and possible cause. History of surgery in neonatal period for correction of congenital anorectal anomalies may be useful.

5.1. Clinically the external anal orifice is patulous without any scar in the perineum and faecal soiling of perianal skin. The impaired sensation in touch or to pin prick implies that the success of the operative repair will not be a satisfied one. Clinical examination may reveal evidence of generalized disorders likely to be responsible for incontinence such as Parkinson's disease, Multiple sclerosis, Dementia or Alzheimer's disease.

5.2. Rectal examination

While doing the rectal examination, the tone of the sphincter can be evaluated by asking the patient to tighten up the anus, and may reveal the defect in the anal sphincter. Malignancy in anorectal region, prolapse rectum, Perianal descends or faecal impaction could be made out in rectal examination.

6. INVESTIGATIONS

Anorectal Physiological tests will define anatomical defects, the quality of anorectal function and identify the neurological defects.

6.1. Anorectal manometry
The resting pressure reflects the function of the internal sphincter and squeeze pressure that of the external sphincter function. The normal resting pressure is 40mm Hg and that of squeeze pressure 80mmHg.

6.2. Electromyography
It will be useful in assessing the degree of conduction defect and help to determine, the presence and location of the residual muscle in patients with congenital anorectal anomalies.

6.3. Pudendal Nerve Terminal Motor Latency (PNTML)
There may be pudendal nerve injury because of prolonged labour in addition to sphincter injury, so PNTML may predict the likelihood of successful repair of sphincter.

PNTML measures the conducting time to the external anal sphincter after the pudental nerve stimulation at the level of ischial spine. This is performed by using a digitally mounded device with stimulating electrode mounted at the fingertip and the recording electrode mounded in the base of the finger. The self-adhesive disposable electrode can be mounted on a gloved finger. The normal Latency is 2.1 ±0.2 minutes. Prolonged latency can occur in pudendal nerve damage in consistent straining conditions like prolapsed rectum, Perianal descent, and prolonged second stage Labour. PNTML predict the success rate of surgery following sphincter repair.

6.4. Endo anal Ultra Sound (EUS)
When endoanal ultra-sonography is done by an experienced sinologist, 100% sensitivity and specificity in identifying internal and external anal

sphincter defect, the morphology of the anal sphincter defect, puborectalis sling, and in female recto vaginal septum can be demonstrated well. Vaginal Endo sonography may demonstrate the status of anterior part of anal sphincter. EUS is a safe procedure, easy to performed and well accepted by the patient.

6.5. Magnetic Resonance Imaging (MRI)

MRI provides more detailed informations about the anatomy of the sphincters.

7. MANAGEMENT FECAL INCONTINENCE:

Most patients with mild to moderate symptoms successfully responded to conservative treatment and this must be considered as first line of treatment.

7.1. Prevention of incontinence

Incontinence due to Iatrogenic should be preventable. Obstetrical injury could be avoided by a more vigorous selection of patients with cephalo pelvic disproportion for elective Caesarean section, by preventing a prolonged a second stage labour, doing episiotomy whenever the sphincter is liable to be damaged by foetal head.

7.2. The colonic, rectal, and anal diseases must be treated appropriately. Many patients know when they are likely to be incontinent and have adjusted their daily activities accordingly.

The aim of bowel management programme is to establish a routine for defecation that is safe, convenient, and dependable. Ideally, the bowel can be re-educated to empty regularly, and at a predictable time.

7.3. Although it is not possible to increase the internal anal sphincter tone by Perianal strengthening exercise, voluntary contraction of the external sphincter, Puborectalis sling and Levator ani muscle, may improve the continence. A simple exercise is, pretending to hold the bowel movement for about 10-15 seconds done for 15 to 20 times a day.

7.4. Many patients with incontinence will know when they are likely to be incontinent and have adjusted their daily pattern of activities accordingly. Bulk laxatives may provide a soft stool of predictable size and consistency and making bowel action more regular.

7.5. Drug therapy

Constipating drugs such as lopramide, lomotil, and codeine are often used in the first line of treatment in faecal incontinence particularly those with loose motion. Lopramide has multiple action.

i. Increases the fluid absorption.

ii. Decreases the mucus secretion.

iii. Alter the stool volume and consistency.

iv. Slowing colonic transit.

v. Increases the internal anal sphincter pressure and enhances the continence.

A topical agent such as 10% phenylnephrine increases internal anal sphincter contraction and thus increases the resting tone. It is more useful in minor soiling associated with decreased resting tone. Suppositories, enema, or rectal irrigation may be used to stimulate evacuation at a time when the patient has easy access to toilet and make them free of soiling for the rest of the day.

A variety of methylcellulose and Psyllium products are available in powder, granules and pills. Cholestyramine and colestipol are resins used to treat bile acid diarrhoea by binding with bile salts in the small intestine. They also alter the absorption of fat-soluble vitamins.

7.6. Adult patients with over flow incontinence and paediatric patients with encopresis present with complaints of faecal incontinence, due to constant seepage of stool from a full rectum. The treatment for both conditions begins with digital disimpaction, colonic cleaning, followed by use of cathartic such as polyethylene glycol preparation.

8. BOWEL MANAGEMENT

The goal of effective bowel management programme is to allow the patient to produce a complete bowel movements at a scheduled time by using an individualised combination of dietary measures, laxative, suppositories, enema or digital evacuation. This approach to bowel dysfunction commonly used in spinal cord injuries and patients with some neurological disorders like multiple sclerosis, congenital disorder(Imperforate anus, spina bifida) decreased rectal sensation, and incomplete evacuation.

9. PHYSIOTHERAPY AND ELECTRICAL STIMULATION

Physiotherapy in the form of pelvic floor exercises may improve residual sphincter function. If the striated muscle contract following Pudendal nerve stimulation, electrical stimulation may be useful in such cases. Even if the contraction is delayed, augmentation of sphincter mechanism may be possible. Repeated simulation of Pelvic floor muscle can enhance the EMG activities in these muscles and improve the sphincter function.

10. ANAL INCONTINENCE PLUG

The anal incontinence plug prevents Trans anal flow of gas and faecal materials. This disposable plug is inserted by the patient and removed manually to evacuate the rectum(fig 14.03).

The Anal Plug is available in two sizes 37 and 45 mm diameter. Patients with reduced or absent anorectal sensitivity have some benefit from the usage of anal plug. The anal plug consists of a cup shaped foam plug with a gauze string for removal. It is wrapped in a clear water-soluble film to keep compact for insertion. This film dissolves on contact with moised rectal mucosa and the plug opens up.

11. BIO FEEDBACK

The Biofeedback therapy is best applied to motivated patient with some ability to voluntarily contact the external anal sphincter and intact rectal sensation (fig 13.02). Using a surface EMG anal probe, the patient can be taught to contract sphincter and levator ani in response to rectal distension. With the help of dense electrical impulses generated by the active muscles were fed back to the patient in the form of audible or visible signals. Several home Biofeedback systems are available.

The three Balloon systems is popular. This device involves measuring internal anal sphincter relaxation and external sphincter contraction with three intra anal balloons while the balloon in the rectum is used to stimulate rectal distension sensation.

12. RADIOFREQUENCY THERAPY (SECCA PROCEDURE)

Radiofrequency (RF) therapy is based on the theory that delivery of radiofrequency energy via an endoanal probe could potentially improve the barrier function of the anal sphincter complex. The SECCA system is designed to deliver temperature controlled Radiofrequency energy into the muscle of the anal canal for the treatment of faecal incontinence. The Radiofrequency energy hand piece is composed of a clear anoscope barrel with four nickel- titanium curved needle electrodes (22 gauge, 6mm in length). The SECCA procedure is a minimally invasive ambulatory one and the patient can return to normal activity within 48 hours. This treatment may be offered a lost resort to a patient for whom there is no alternative except faecal diversion in the form of colostomy.

13. SURGICAL TREATMENT:

The two primary method of surgical treatment for anal incontinence are available.

i. Direct repair of a localised sphincter defect.
ii. Repair designed to supplement the sphincter mechanism.

The most common indication for surgery in anal incontinence is post obstetrical injury. Occult sphincter defects are extremely common after vaginal delivery particularly when forceps are applied for delivery of the child. The symptom of faecal incontinence worsens with long-term follow up.

13.1. Post anal repair

Park originally described post anal repair in 1975 for patients with idiopathic faecal incontinence. Now it is also done for incontinence associated with rectal prolapse and descending Perianal syndrome. The aim of this procedure is to restore the anorectal angle and lengthening of the anal canal by placating the muscles of pelvic floor. The sphincter pressure and anal canal mucosal electro sensitivity is improved post operatively along with anal canal sensation. The operation increases the length of the high-pressure zone in the anal canal and there is significant improvement in resting and squeezing pressure.

A posterior curved incision is made in the Perianal region and the dissection is done in the intersphinteric plane. The anal canal is lifted forward with its surrounding sphincter away from the external sphincter and from the sides up to the level of Puborectalis. The limbs of the Puborectalis sling are then opposed by a series of interrupted sutures. The external sphincter is finally sutured. Miller et al describe anterior approach for sphincter placation and levator plasty in 1989.

13.2. PERINEORRAPHY

When the incontinence is due to third obstetrical laceration of the perineum, perineorraphy is undertaken. The scar tissues are excised; the defect in the vagina is closed. The Puborectalis sling and the anal sphincter muscles are sutured individually.

13.3. Sphincter repair

The sphincter repair treatments include excision of skin scar and define the sphincter muscle with preservation of the fibrous ends for securing the sutures. The skin wound may be left open or partially sutured. Three standard operations for repairing the injured sphincter are

i. Opposition.

ii. Overlapping.

iii. Placation.

Identification of the cut ends of the sphincter can be made by muscle stimulation.

Techniques

The mucosa of the anal canal and lower rectum is mobilized and opposed with absorbable suture material. The divided ends of the sphincter are dissected with special care to avoid excessive mobilization and excessive removal of fibrous scar tissues. This allows for repair of normally vascularised and innervated sphincter mechanism by an overlapping technique. Mattress suture with fine non absorbable suture incorporating fibrous scar tissue adherent to the mobilized edges of the sphincter to the underlying healthy muscle ensure tight anal canal. It is not necessary to identify the external and internal sphincter separately. The sphincter mass is identified, freed from the fibrous scar and sutured. It may appear at first, the circumference of the anal canal is reduced by about half, but gradually stretched in due course.

Early repair procedures for segmental sphincter defect in the form of direct end-to-end suture of the sphincter have difficulty in identifying the muscle ends and hold them together. This may be the reason for failure in some cases. Per operative muscle fibre stimulation and overlapping suture technique improve the success rate.

13.4. Muscle transposition (supplementary muscle for sphincter mechanism)

When too much of muscle tissue (sphincter), has been lost as the result of trauma, the effective reconstruction may not be possible. In these situations surgical reconstruction designed to create a supplementary muscle may have some merits. This can be done for failed sphincter repair. Gluteus Maximus, gracilis, adductor longus, and Sartorius are the muscles used substitute to anal sphincter.

13.4.1. Gluteo plasty

The advantages of using gluteus Maximus muscle for Sphincteroplasty are:

i. Single proximal innervations.

ii. Proximity to the anal canal.

iii. Large bulky muscle (lower 10% of both gluteus muscles are used).

iv. Buttocks contraction is a standard response to impending incontinence.

13.4.2. Graciloplasty

The muscle length, its constant proximal innervations by the obsturator nerve, and dominant proximal vascular supply by profunda femoris make it suitable for this procedure (fig 14.01). Because the gracilis muscle consists of predominantly of type II, the transposed muscle appears more to mimic circular stenosis, a kind of living 'Thiersch's wire', than to constitute a dynamic substitute. Once the muscle is transposed and wrapped around the anus, and encircling with muscle tissue and not the tendon, which is fixed to ischial tuberosity.

13.4.3. Dynamic Graciloplasty

The finding that fatigue prone, fast twitch muscle fibres (type II) can be converted to fatigue resistant, slow twitch muscle fibres (type I) by continuous low frequency simulation, led to the evolution of dynamic Graciloplasty. This procedure involves the transposition of gracilis muscle and implantation of an electrical stimulation device consisting of electrodes and an impulse generator. After the Graciloplasty technique is over, the neuro stimulation device is implanted simultaneously or as two-stage operation.

Two different techniques have been used. i. Direct neural stimulation with placement of electrodes around the nerve. ii. Neuro Stimulator with intermusclar electrodes placed through the muscle close to the entrance of the nerve. In both techniques, the electrodes either are connected to a pulse generator placed in a subcutaneous or sub fascial pocket in the lower abdomen.

13.5. Sub mucosal injection of ACYST

Acyst is comprised of carrier water and Beta- D glucon and pyrolitic carbon beads measuring 212 - 500 vm. The Compound is injected into the sub mucosa of the lower rectum and upper anal canal just above the level of dentate line. The mechanism of action is that the compound bulks up the anal canal by increasing the sub mucosa and 'plugging 'the anal canal. In addition to the increased bulk, may allow for improved sensation and discrimination.

13.6. Artificial Bowel Sphincter (ABS)

An artificial bowel sphincter is an implantable, fluid filled, solid silicone elastomeric devise. It consists of three components, a cuff, a control pump with septum and a pressure-regulating balloon, attached to each other with kink resistant tubing. The ABS stimulates the normal sphincter function by opening and closing the anal canal at the control of the patient(fig 14.04).

The occlusive cuff is implanted around a segment of anal canal and when inflated it occludes the anal canal by applying pressure circumferentially around the anal canal. The pressure-regulating balloon is implanted in the perivesical space and controls the amount of pressure exerted by the occlusion cuff. The control pump is implanted in the soft tissue of the scrotum or labia. The upper part of the control pump contains the register and valve needed to transfer fluid in and from the cuff. The patient squeezes and relaxes to transfer fluid within the device.

13.7. Sacral Nerve Stimulation (SNS)

Sacral nerve stimulation is adopted for the treatment of faecal incontinence in patients with functional deficits of anal sphincter but no morphological deficits in which conservative treatment had failed. The rationale applying SNS as a treatment of faecal incontinence is based on the observation of its effect on Anorectal continence in urological patients (increased anorectal angulation and increased anal canal closure pressure) and on anatomical consideration – dual peripheral nerve supply of the pelvic floor muscle that covers these functions.

13.8. Faecal diversion

A temporary faecal diversion is done in selected cases after sphincter repair (colostomy or Ileostomy). When the surgical treatment is failed on repeated occasions and when other methods of control of soiling is not possible creation of stoma will improve the quality of life. The stoma can be managed by routine ways.

CHAPTER 12

BACTERIAL SYNERGISIC INFECTION

Bacterial synergistic infection is the soft tissue infection presents a variety of clinical and pathological entities and is characterised by i. Tissue necrosis. ii. Rapid progression. iii. Lack of frank suppuration. iv. Systemic toxicity.

1. BACTERIOLOGY AND PATHOGENESIS

The infection is due to Polymicrobial Synergistic infection. Typically, the organisms consist of facultative Streptococcus and Gram-negative anaerobic rods. Highly virulent Gram-negative aerobes such as P. aeroginosa and certain Streptococcus species such as St. Pyogenes. It can be caused by mono microbial organisms.

2. BACTERIAL SYNERGISM

Bacterial Synergism is defined as an effect on a host found in the presence of two or more organisms, but the effect on the host not seen with either organism alone. The mechanism of bacterial synergism maybe:

i. One organism may facilitates transmission to colonization of the host by second organism.

ii. One organism may attenuated local or systemic host resistance, allowing invasion by second organism.

iii. One organism may increase the virulence of another.

iv. One organism may provide growth factor for another organism.

3. THE BACTERIAL SYNERGISTIC INFECTION IS CLASSIFIED AS

i. Maloney's gangrene.
ii. Necrotizing Fasciitis.
iii. Clostridia Myonecrosis.
iv. Fournier's Gangrene. A condition of combination of all above.

Bacterial Synergistic infection It can arise after abdominal, pelvic or Perianal surgery. Anaerobic cellulitis may arise spontaneously particularly when it involves abdomen the development of these severe infection, debilitating hosts (elderly, diabetic, immuno-suppressed individuals) and introduction of one or more organisms into the soft tissue.

3.1. Maloney's synergistic gangrene (Cutaneous Synergistic gangrene)

The infection is characterized by a tender erythematosis area with central purpuric zone which leads to gangrene. The causative organisms are micro aerophlic non-haemolytic Streptococcus and St. Aureus. The causative organism may vary according to the site of infection. For instance if it arises in association with anorectal diseases then colonic bacteria will be responsible. In most cases, numerous species of both aerobic and anaerobic are found.

3.2. Necrotizing fasciitis

It is a subcutaneous infection of mixed bacterial origin due to Gram positive cocci (both aerobic and anaerobic) and Gram negative bacilli. Cutaneous signs are often absent, but dish water drainage from the wound is a classical finding.

3.3. Clostridia Myonecrosis

It is the gas gangrenes which rapidly progressive infection of skeletal muscle usually due to Clostridium Perfringens. The onset is rapid with severe local pain, oedema, dishwater discharge, and crepitus with systemic toxaemia.

3.4. Fournier's gangrene

It is a synergistic bacterial infection. It has components of cutaneous gangrene, necrotizing fasciitis and Myonecrosis. Jean Alfred Fournier first described the condition in 1883.

Not all Perianal infections results in necrosis and gangrene. Some special conditions must exist to allow the infection that eventually leads to Fournier's gangrene. In most cases there is deficiencies in the immune system. Local conditions like relative hypoxia may initiate the infective process. The infective organisms must be sufficient and appropriate bacteria, like Gram-positive aerobic and anaerobic cocci and Gram-negative bacilli is essential.

4. PATHOGENESIS

4.1. The port of entry is from gastrointestinal tract or genitourinary tract. Anorectal abscess or fistula is the most common gastrointestinal source. Urethral stricture and instrumentation with subsequent infection of peri urethral gland is the most common cause of genitourinary source. Virtually all patients have demonstrable port of organisms particularly perianal infection. Delay in treating the infection in the initial stage is the most important contributing factor.

4.2. The skin necrosis and crepitating occurs in early. The infection typically starts in the scrotum or penile skin. Swelling and associated fever and chillness may be the clinical presentation. There may be septic shock. The affected area may be acutely tender, however once gangrene sets in, the skin become anaesthetic, as the result of destruction of subcutaneous sensory nerves. Spontaneous drainage of brown watery (dish water) discharge may occur with characteristic feculent odour.

4.3. Randell in 1920 described the full-blown Perianal gangrene as follows. "When the scrotum is involved, the skin, subcutaneous tissue, dartos facia and all structure of its wall, come away in a stringy, fetid mass. The testis bared to their vaginalis, hang suspended by their cords, shamefully exposed, though remarkably free from gangrene and obvious to their new surroundings (or possibly should I say, lack of surroundings) and can be handled freely without causing the slightest discomfort".

5. DIAGNOSIS

These infections are often difficult to diagnose initially because the disease process extends in the deep soft tissues without causing extensive external skin changes. Eventually, however, the skin with affected area develop colour changes, blisters may form, crepitation can be detected due to gas forming organisms. The infection initially causes vascular thrombosis, then subcutaneous tissue necrosis and eventually dermal gangrene. The patient may develop septic shock.

5.1. In case of gastrointestinal origin, Gram-negative bacteria and Bacteriods predominate. Origin from genitourinary tract, E. coli and Streptococcus species are most common. In cases related to trauma, break in the skin integrity, and causes infection, Staphylococcus and Streptococcus species are most common organisms. In gangrene associated with haematological malignancy, Pseudomonas is the common pathogen.

5.2. It is now possible, by using gas liquid chromatography to distinguish very rapidly (30minutes to 1 hour) between anaerobic and aerobic infection. In the specimen of pus, anaerobic bacteria are recognized by the production of some fatty acid. Isolation of anaerobic bacteria is improved if fluid samples are sent in capped syringes.

5.3. Scrotal ultra sonography. In selected cases scrotal ultra-sonogram may be useful in distinguish Fournier's gangrene from epididymo - orchitis and torsion testis. The sonological findings with Fournier gangrene are

i. Thickening and oedema of the scrotal skin.

ii. Subcutaneous air in the scrotum.

iii. Normal Testis and epididymis.

6. TREATMENT

The treatment is considered in four important aspects.

i. Broad Spectrum antibiotics.

ii. Wide surgical debridement.

iii. Systemic support.

iv. Wound management and delayed closure.

6.1. Antibiotics

Initial Gram staining is of value in detecting the presence of Gram positive or Gram negative alone or in combination. This enable the best antibiotics to be started. The important in the management of patients is detection and isolation of organisms from the source of infection as well as from the blood, so that specific antibiotics can be started. Broad-spectrum antibiotics are essential. The selected antibiotics should provide coverage against Gram-positive cutaneous flora, enteric and genitourinary Gram-negative bacteria and anaerobes. Ampicillin, gentamycin, and clindamycin provide adequate coverage until the culture reports are available. Penicillin G is recommended for clostridia infection.

6.2. Incision and wide surgical debridement

The important aspect of treatment is incision, wide excision and a combination of antibiotics. Vigorous surgical excision and debridement of all nonviable tissues are imperative. Debridement must be radical and should be continued until the skin and subcutaneous tissues cannot be separated from live fascia. Pus is to be drained as early as possible and re drain in as frequent as necessary. The same is true for the debridement of necrotic tissues. Gangrene may develop in the cut surface of the wound within 24-48 hours (die again). Irrigation of the wound with hydrogen peroxide should be done frequently. Colostomy may be needed in some cases to prevent wound infection from faecal contamination.

6.3. Systemic Support

Systemic support includes fluid resuscitation, correction of electrolyte and acid base abnormalities, hypoxia, and treatment of underlying co-morbid conditions. Blood glucose level to be measured and hyperglycaemia is treated with intravenous insulin. However, these measures should not significantly delay surgical intervention. The timing of surgery is critical and the patient should be resuscitated adequately to the optimum level as early as possible.

6.4. The critically ill patients can be considered as either Immuno compromised host or the victim of an exaggerated inflammatory response. The therapeutic implication is often diametrically opposite. Immuno compromised host has to have therapeutics strategies as nonspecific stimulation of Immune system with levamisole, systemic administration of pro inflammatory drugs like cytokine interferon. In exaggerated inflammatory response, the antagonist of immuno suppressive mediator such as Prostaglandin is given.

6.5. Hyperbaric oxygen therapy

Hyperbaric oxygen therapy theoretically works by increasing oxygen tension within the tissue, thereby creating an environment poorly suitable for anaerobic growth.

7. WOUND MANAGEMENT

7.1. Frequent dressing changing, as often as 4-6 hourly in the early postoperative period is required. Saline soaked gauze is as effective as many antibacterial solutions and promotes epithelialisation. Dressing changes may provide debridement of small amount of necrotic tissues but repeat surgical would debridement is often necessary.

7.2. Once the healing granulation tissue is formed in the wound depending up on their size and location, some wounds may be allowed to close by second intention. However, others may need operative closure. In most instances, split skin graft may provide good covering for the wound. Local flap reconstruction may occasionally be needed. If the testis needs skin cover, it may be necessary to place the testis in subcutaneous packet in the thigh.

7.3. Place of Honey in wound management

The organisms commonly associated with bacteria synergistic Infection is sensitive to microbial action of honey. The antimicrobials effect of honey lies with physical property of solute concentration phenomenon. It has been proved that no organism grow in the media in which more than 30% concentration of honey present due to hyper osmolarity as the result of hyperosmolar concentration. It causes rapid absorption of oedema fluid from soggy, weeping wounds. The viscosity of the honey is larger, it forms a physical barrier, and it prevents bacterial colonization.

The improved monitoring techniques have led a more rational treatment with a consequent reduction in mortality. Resuscitation and surgical drainage may be more important for successful outcomes. Delayed primary closure, skin grafting and other reconstructive procedure are often required. The ultimate outcome is determined by the underlying pathology, the integrity of the host mechanism and the presence of associated diseases.

CHAPTER 13

PERIANAL HIDRADINITIS SUPPURATION (PHS)

Sweat glands are of two types, eccrin and apocrine. Eccrin are distributed diffusely over the body and regulate the body temperature by producing sweat. Apocrine glands are in limited distribution, larger than the eccrin and extend deeper into the dermis. The apocrine glands ducts open not on to the skin but into a pilosebaceous orifice. Therefore, they are limited hair bearing part of the anal region, in the axilla, groin, areola, sub mammary fold, periumbilical area and scalp. Their secretions are thick and melodious. Hidradinitis supportiva is a chronic recurrent fulminatory process involving the apocrine glands.

1. GENERAL CONSIDERATION

Apocrine secretion is adrenergically controlled, but the exact mechanism by which the catecholamine reach the gland is not well established. It is suggested that the first phase of secretions, production within the apocrine tubules and the second phase is expulsion of the secretion to the surface by contraction of Myoepithelelial cells surrounding the duct.

1.2. Apocrine gland infection

Hidradinitis suppuration has high chances of chronicity. A combination of acute infection with multifocal suppuration and abscess formation as well as chronic scarring and fistula formation is the commonest clinical presentation. The process may extend into the inter gluteal cleft or perianal region. The condition is not life threatening but annoying and causes significant work absence.

1.3. It occurs in oily skin, Endocrine disorder persons, such as diabetes mellitus, and obesity individuals. Nicotine from smoking stimulates the secretion in apocrine glands.

2. PATHOGENESIS

2.1. The hidradinitis suppuration usually starts after puberty, coincident with activation of the apocrine secretion. Androgens are associated with increased keratinisation of the skin. That may predispose keratin occlusion of the duct.

Once occlusion to the duct occurs, a chain of events takes place.. Stasis of the secretion in the gland ductules, infection and bacterial proliferation, suppuration, ruptures into the skin, surrounding subcutaneous tissue, multiple epithelial tracts, and fibrosis of the skin. Once the gland got infected due to ductal obstruction, the surrounding inflammation predispose to obstruction in the neighbouring glands and thus spreading the disease. Dermal scaring and chronic sinuses are the result of recurrent inflammation. There is progressive destruction of the skin architecture with multiple painful discharging sinuses on hair bearing area. Secondary infection causes fibrosis, which destroys the gland unit.

2.2. The destroyed apocrine glands coalesce to form sub cutaneous abscess and discharge through more than one site resulting is extensive subcutaneous sinuses that rarely heals without treatment. Eventually chronic inflammatory process results in significant fibrosis and scaring of the involved skin forming the characteristic ' pit- like' scar. The damaged pilosebaceous unite eventually coalesce to form network of chronically draining subcutaneous abscess and sinuses. The sinuses and fistula are usually superficial. Subcutaneous tunnelling involving extensive area of skin is common. Differentiation from perianal Crohn's disease may be difficult and both may co-exist. If untreated there is long time risk of malignant transformation into Squamous cell carcinoma over a period of 20to 30 years.

3. THE BACTERIAL FLORA

The bacteria involved in hidradinitis are inconsistent and unpredictable. Staphylococcus epidermis, E.coli, klebsiella, Proteus, Alpha streptococcus, Anaerobic bacteria, and Diphtherioid were cultured from the wound swabs of these patients. Some others reported Chlamydia trachomatis is also responsible.

4. CLINICAL PRESENTATION

The clinical presentation is characterized by remission and relapsing. Pain leading to unbearable to sit down, swelling and purulent discharges from multiple openings and secondary skin infection. As the disease worsen, the extend of skin involvement increases with areas of acute inflammation and abscess co-existing with areas of chronic discharging sinuses.

4.1. With each recurrence

The subcutaneous cavities tend to be larger. The result is an indurated, fibrotic subcutaneous cavities and sinus tracts, the extend of which can be highly variable. Some patients are affected in limited regions with mild disease and others are affected by extensive involvements at multiple sites, cycles of remission and relapse are typical. Each episode causes distressing pain and embarrassing foul smelling discharge.

4.2. Perianal Hidradinitis Suppuration (PHS)

This is defined as inflammation of sweat glands forming pus at perianal region. Some says it is infection of apocrine gland. Most of the cases are chronic recurrent disease. This has to be differentiated from Fistula, Pyoderma, Squamous cell Carcinoma, Crohn's disease,

Lympho granuloma venereum, Perianal Tuberculosis and rarely from Actinomycosis.

4.3. The aggressive form of hidradinitis surpurativa known as Follicular Occlusive Tetrad. This is comprised of:

i. Hidradinitis.

ii. Peri folliculitis.

iii. Nodular cystic acne vulgarise.

iv. Pilonidal sinus.

This condition though rare, may cause severe anorectal sepsis. The Perianal lesions may be extensive with involvement of the scrotum, groin, and buttock, with extensive fibrosis.

Acne conglomata is a severe manifestation of acne involving the chest, back, and buttock and small purulent nodules are the features. Peri folliculitis capitis is a similar condition involving inflammatory and purulent nodules on the scalp. Due to chronic sepsis there may be bone marrow depression resulting in anaemia or may affect nutritional status causing hypo protinemia.

5. DIAGNOSIS

The diagnosis of extensive perianal and Perianal lesions are usually straightforward. When limited to an acute abscess or a few discharging sinuses, it is difficult to diagnose. The diagnosis of limited perianal or Perianal lesion is one of exclusion because the disease has no pathonomic clinical or histological features.

5.1. Probing of the sinus under anaesthesia may show their origin and depth. Fistulous tract opening at dentate line are not due to hidradinitis. However, the fistula due to hidradinitis, the internal opening is 2/3 rd of the way, the skin lined part of anal canal. Sinuses that extend deeply into the ischiorectal fossa or Para rectal space are very unlikely due to hidradinitis.

5.2. Differential Diagnosis

In extensive disease, the diagnosis is quite obvious. Sometimes the following conditions to be considered for exclusion:

i. Multiple fistula in ano.

ii. Perianal tuberculosis.

iii. Lymphoma granuloma Venerium.

iv. Crohn's disease.

v. Actinomycosis.

vi. Pyoderma.

vii. Pilonidal sinus.

viii. Carcinoma.

6. TREATMENT

There are several methods of treatment.

i. Non operative management.

ii. Simple incision and drainage.

iii. Un roofing of multiple tracts.

iv. Wide local excision with or without skin graft.

v. Marsupialisation of the excised area.

vi. Wide excision with hydrocolloid or hydro gel dressing.

vii. Incision and drainage followed by irradiation.

6.1. Non operative management

In obesity, individual weight reduction advises to be given. Avoid tight fitting clothing and advice loose fitting cotton clothing particularly under wears. Advice antiseptic body care. Culture and sensitivity test from discharge should be done before selecting the antibiotics. The antibiotics may be given systemically or locally as ointment. The effect of antibiotics cannot be predicted in spite of the sensitivity test because of fibrosis along the tract by chronic infection the antibiotics may not reach the target area in effect concentrations.

6.2. Operative Treatment

INDICATIONS

i. Symptomatic disease. Acute or sub-acute suppuration or abscess.

ii. Extensive area of involvement.

iii. Refractory to conservative treatment.

iv. Suspicions of malignancy.

6.3. If lay open is chosen, care should be taken to incise all extensions, trimming the edges of the sinuses or tracts leaving the fibrous tract intact. Lay open is indicated when the disease is superficial and are more nuisances.

Un roofing involves probing and explore all sinuses tracts and fistulas, completely removing the roof of all tracts, curetting the tracts and leaving the floor intact to aid in closure by secondary intention. The technique is somewhat tedious and time consuming but leaves island of epithelium from which regeneration occurs rapidly. Un roofing especially valuable in extensive perianal disease.

Limited local excision is indicated if involvement of the disease is in limited area. Primary closure of the wound is done. Local excision is associated with a high rate of recurrence. The risk of local recurrence in perianal lesions is comparatively less.

6.4. Wide Excision

Extensive disease causing significant symptoms needs excision. Once the disease process has become chronic and extensive most surgeons recommend excision of the affected area of apocrine glands bearing skin 1 to 2cm beyond visible evidence of the disease to minimize the risk of recurrence. The affected area should be excised down to normal subcutaneous area to ensure adequate removal of all apocrine glands.

The wound can be managed by one of the several ways including primary closure if possible, split skin graft coverage, advancement flap cover or healing by secondary intension. Recurrence is related to the adequacy of resection and severity of the disease, not the selected method of wound closure. For wide excision Co2 laser or harmonic scalpel have been used. Extensive area as the result of wide excision may need faecal diversion in the form of colostomy.

6.5. Marsupialisation

Suturing of the wound edges to the fibrous base of the wound to avoid retraction of the skin edges and allow for easier wound care and proper quick healing.

Controversy still exists regarding the optimal surgical treatment. Factors that influence is the extent of surgery includes the site affected, the extent of the disease and whether is acute or chronic presentation. 25% of recurrence of the disease are due to the disease developing in a new area. The risk of recurrence after a "successful "treatment is 30 to 50%. The patient should be informed of the need for meticulous hygiene.

7. Hidradinitis may coexist with perianal Crohn's fistula in patients with severe rectal Crohn's disease. The consequences of the mistaken diagnosis can be significant, as it will influence the result of the surgical treatment. So be aware of combination of perianal hidradinitis and Crohn's disease. Squamous cell carcinoma may develop in long standing cases.

8. HORMONAL TREATMENT

Androgen level thought to play a role in disease activity. It can be reduced with steroid by suppressing the hypothalamus pituitary axis. A systemic gonadotropin releasing hormone (Leuprolide) has also been used to inhibit the axis. Anti-androgen Cyproteron Acetate available in Europe has encouraging success rate.

CHAPTER 14

ANAL CONDYLOMATA

The condylomata are ano genital warts, of hyper keratic, cauliflower like, solitary or multiple skin lesions. They are caused by sexually transmitted disease of squamous epithelium, with highly contagious Human Papilloma Virus (HPV). The genital warts or condylomata accumulatas are on increasingly prevalent condition that represents the most commonly encountered venereal disease in surgical practice. It is often found in homosexual men. Not all condylomata are acquired by sexual contact. The virus may present in the skin and can be transmitted by hands.

1.1. CAUSATIVE FACTORS

In 1968 intra cellular viral particles, a papova DNA virus, in human genital warts tissues was demonstrated. The etiological agent is found out to be Human Papilloma Virus (HPV). The papova DNA Virus is the only virus known to produce tumour in human. It is found most often in homosexual man. The association with anal intercourse varies from 46-to95percentage in the reported series. So the presence of anal warts does not necessarily imply that the patient engage in anal sex practice. The virus anti genically, Bio chemically, and immunologically distinct from Virus of common warts, veruga vulgarise.

1.2. There are more than 60 types of HPV. Those associated with anal condyloma are usually HPV6, 11, and 2. HPV6 and11 are typically associated will benign diseases. HPV 16 and18 are associated with cervical and intra epithelial neoplasia, which may progress in to invasive

Squamous cell carcinoma, particularly in homosexual men (MSM). HPV 16 and 18 are dominant oncogenic type with invasive Squamous cell carcinoma of the anus and perianal region.

1.3. Immuno compromised patients in general have a high evidence of condyloma and ano genital neoplasm than the general population. Condyloma accumulatas are frequent among HIV positive and AIDS patients. Missed lesions may act as a reservoir of infection in the anal canal. HPV may be dormant within the cells for months and even years. The exact anal donor of infection therefore cannot be determined with certainty.

2. PATHOLOGY

2.1. Histologically condylomata are squamous cell papilloma. Microscopic features are:

i. papillomatous, Hyper keratinisation,

ii. Acanthotic and presence of clear cells within the Acanthotic epithelium.

iii. The hyperkerotic Acanthotic lesions maintains epithelial maturation towards the surface. It has characteristic koilocytosis peri nuclear cytoplasmic vacuolization in conjunction with nuclear irregularity.

iv. Low-grade dysplasia (AIN I) to high-grade Dysplasia (AIN III) increasing epithelial disorganization, loss of maturation, increased cellularity to the surface can be demonstrated histological examination.

2.2. Buschke Loewenstein giant condylomata

These lesions are large, expansive, verucous growth with invasive squamous cell carcinoma (verucous carcinoma). They are locally destructive growth pattern with high risk for local recurrence but low tendency to metastasize. They are locally invasive without penetrating lymphatic or blood vessels. This type of condyloma is associated with HPV type 6 and 11.

2.3. Subclinical HPV infection in the perineum or anal region may appear as a flat, non-raised white epithelium after applying 5% acetic acid (acetowhite). Biopsy of these area shows HPV infection in 78% and intra epithelial dysplasia was noted in acetowhite epithelium in 8% of cases. HPV appears to be auto inoculable, which explains the tendency of warts to recur after treatment. The incubation period may be as short as 4 weeks but may be a year or more.

2.4. Condyloma accumulatas may found as associated lesions in the penis, distal urethra, vulva and vagina, anal canal and distal 1to 2 cm of rectum. So clinical examination to be done in genital organs. Proctoscopic examination is necessary in all cases to exclude intra anal extension of the lesion.

Malignant transformation of giant condylomata accumulatas has been reported. Verruca carcinoma is considered low grade, well-differentiated type of squamous cell carcinoma.

3. CLINICAL PRESENTATION

3.1. The lesion is more common in sexually active age period. The male female radio of the disease is 9: 2. Itching and difficult in cleaning, are the common complaints. Increasing in size and Bleeding even for minor trauma are other complaints. Pain is not the symptom in anal warts and they are often asymptomatic, therefore it may lead to delay in starting the treatment.

3.2. Based upon the clinical presentation condylomata are classified as

i. Condyloma plana.
ii. Condyloma accuminata.
iii. Condyloma gigantica (Buschke Loewenstein).

The patient may present with large exophytic warts. Due to confluence of the warts, the lesion may look like a carpet. Sometimes it may appear as scattered warts. In Male 13 to 30 % of anal warts have associated penile warts and 70 to 85% of patients with external warts in the perineum have extension of the lesion in to the anal canal.

4. DIFFERENTIAL DIAGNOSIS

i. Condyloma lata. The lesion is smooth and rather flattened than condyloma accumulata and there may be other signs of syphilis such as macula papular rashes or snail tract ulcers. The lesion is indurated and weeping mass containing numerous

ii. Spirochetes which can be easily seen under dark ground illumination microscope.

iii. Squamous cell carcinoma. Differentiation between anal condyloma and malignancy may be possible only by total excision biopsy. So excised mass of the condyloma must be subjected to Histopathological examination.

iv. Anal intracellular neoplasia (AIN). Anal dysplasia and carcinoma in situ (CIS) are considered precancerous to the development of invasive squamous cell carcinoma of the anus. These lesions are collectively referred as Anal Intracellular Neoplasia (AIN).

v. Condyloma in relation to HIV.

vi. There is increasing evidence of anal condyloma in HIV population and there is also evidence that they are more aggressive lesions, with more incidences of recurrence, dysplasia and squamous cell carcinoma.

5. TREATMENT

The treatments of the condylomata have taken numerous forms. As is usually the case, when multiple treatments are recommended, none of this work particularly well and no one treatment is satisfactory.

5.1. Chemical agents

5.1.1. Podophyllin

Podophyllin is a resin extracted from the roots of May apple plants. The active agent Podophyllo toxin is an anti-mitotic agent. Podophyllin with Tincture Benzoin 10-20% solution is applied with cotton wool swabs on a slick. The solution is allowed in contact with the lesion for 5 to10 minutes and then it is washed off. The process to be repeated weekly for about 3 months. It is often quite irritating to the surrounding normal anoderm with repeated local and systemic toxicity as well as theoretical oncogenic potentials. These features limit its use for internal anal condyloma. Application of petroleum gel to the normal anoderm surrounding the warts before podophyllin application may limit its local toxicity. Purified Podophyllo toxin (Podofitox) can be self-administered to the perianal lesions. It has a higher therapeutic index than podophyllin itself. The reported complications of podophyllin include severe necrosis, scarring and fistula formation.

5.1.2. Tri chloroacetic acid or Bichloroacetic acid

These cause tissue sloughing but are much less expensive than podophyllin. They require neutralization by Sodium bicarbonate. At least four applications are needed. The result is like that of Podophyllin. Each application kills only superficial few cell layers of the warts and multiple applications are required over a short time to keep the warts from growing faster than the treatment destroying it. Bichloroacetic acid has less systemic effects.

5.2. Chemotherapeutic agents

5.2.1. 5- fluorouracil (5FU)

5% cream of 5FU is applied for 3-7 days. 5 FU with Salicylic acid preparation (Soleoderm) is also used. This treatment often causes intolerable discomfort to the patients. The greatest value of 5 FU may be to prevent recurrence after successful eradication, especially in immuno compromised patients.

5.2.2. Bleomycin

Bleomycin is both antibiotics and anti-tumour agent. Topical injection of Bleomycin 0.1 ml of solution containing 1mg |ml Bleomycin into the base of all lesions every 3-4 weeks over a variable period.

6. IMMUNO THERAPY

Immuno therapy is based upon the concept vaccinating the patients against their own virus. At least 5 grams of excised tissue from the patient is required to prepare the vaccine.

6.1. Interferon

Interferon is proteins with antiviral, anti-tumour and Immuno modulation action that can restore natural killer cells activity. Interferon Alpha and gamma are available for clinical use. It can be used for topical and systemic and intralesional therapy. It is contra indicated in patients with cardiac and renal failures. Adjuvant topical therapy has a real place is current management.

6.2. Imiquimod

This Immuno modulator is a topical agent. When applied locally release endogenous Cytokinin such as interferon. Available as 5% cream and it has activities against genital condyloma. It has to be applied three times a week for 16 weeks. It has minimal ano dermal irritation.

7. SURGICAL TREATMENT

The available surgical treatments are
i.   Cryotherapy.
ii. Diathermy excision.
iii. Laser destruction.
iv. Scissors excision.
v.   Wide excision.

7.1. CRYOTHERAPY

Cry probe is be applied by using nitrous oxide gas or liquid nitrogen. Small lesions can be treated with cryotherapy.

7.2. Diathermy excision

It can be done under local, spinal, or general anaesthesia. Fine tipped diathermy probe is used to avoid excess of skin removal in the pedicle of the warts. Excessive skin loss must be avoided as this may lead to scarring and stenosis at the anal margin. Electro coagulation causes first and 2nd degree burns of condyloma bearing anoderm in using a diathermy. For small lesions the probe is applied over the warts.

7.3. Laser destruction

In view of the high cost of the laser equipment and the risk of fumes in HIV patients, laser treatment is used only in limited places.

7.4. Scissors excision

The base of the warts are infiltrated with 1 in 300,000 adrenaline solution to lift the lesions from the surrounding normal skin and reduce the blood loss. Using fine pair of scissors and dissecting forceps each lesion is excised from the base. It may take a long time for large, and multiple lesions.

7.5. Wide excision

Wide excision is indicated in giant anal condyloma,and lesions with Histopathological evidence of in-situ malignant lesions.

8. RECURRENT CONDYLOMA

Recurrence in majority of cases depends upon the extent of the lesions before treatment. Recurrence within months is likely due to residual virus in the anoderm. Condyloma recurrence in 67% of patients with Biopsy shows HPV but only in 9% of those without residual virus. The belief that the condyloma recurrence is the persistent anodermal HPV after local wart destruction leads to adjuvant HPV treatment with the hope of reducing the recurrence chances. The site of excision is injected with 20 million units of Interferon. The other agents like Imiquimod are under trial.

As already stated, the various types of treatment recommended for anal warts, one to be selected based on size of the lesion, the number of lesions and the suspicions of malignancy. Biopsy of the excised specimen is possible by scissors treatment. Diathermy excision is the main stay in the suspected malignant lesions. The needlepoint cautery tip is more precise when diathermy is used. When new warts are seen after surgical excision, 5 FU cream of 5% can be applied.

CHAPTER 15

ANORECTAL LESIONS IN HIV PATIENTS

Human immunodeficiency virus (HIV) and its inevitable consequences of Acquired Immuno Deficiency Syndrome (AIDS) is a major public health problem throughout the world. Homosexual and bisexual patients with AIDS tend to develop different manifestations of AIDS. HIV associated Anorectal lesions are common in HIV positive who have Men sex with Men (MSM). The treatment option with Highly Active Anti-Viral Treatment (HAAT) has dramatically changed the previously universal fatal. HIV infection such as an opportunistic infection, and HIV associated tumours (lymphoma and Kaposi's sarcoma) have decreased since 1994. Yet the incidence of Anorectal problems have not changed, dysplasia, and anal cancer are on risk. The unprotected anal intercourse appears to be primarily responsible for majority of the problems. As the incidence of AIDS increases, it is important that all physicians to be able to recognize and appropriate management of the Anorectal manifestations of AIDS. HIV positive state or AIDS is important for the protection of treating surgeons and staffs of the team. CD4 counts less than 200 cells/ul is defined as AIDS irrespective of the presence of symptoms or other illnesses.

HIV diagnosis is no more death sentence. People taking treatment survive for decades with the disease. Injectable treatment consisting of Cabotegravir and Rilpiuirine in combination, inhibit the different parts of the virus.

1.1. Incidence

Anorectal lesions in patients with AIDS has occurred in 5.9 to 34%. Although there is large variety of anal diseases associated with HIV positive populations, anal condyloma and anal ulceration make up the vast majority. Cellular immuno deficiency may alter the presentation, diagnosis, or treatment. Genital ulceration secondary to sexually transmitted diseases (STD) actually enhances the transmission of HIV.

In spite of Highly Active Anti-Retroviral, Treatment (HAART) the incidence of Anorectal problems have not changed and anal dysplasia and cancer are on the risk. The original risk of unprotected anal sex appears to be primarily responsible for the majority of the problems.

1.2. Ano receptive intercourse with its attended risk factors for STD and HIV infection is not limited to the male but also occur in female who engage in ano receptive intercourse but the incidence of HIV infection is less in female comparing male.

2. PATHOGENESIS

2.1. The mucosal sheds from the rectum contains immunoglobulin A that traps foreign antigens and expels them with stool, preventing them from reaching the anal crypt cells. The cellular immunity is controlled by the Langerhans dendrite cells, which communicate with T cells through a complicated mechanism, identify foreign cells. This allows the entire complement of cell mediated immunity to destroy that, which is alien.

2.2. The mechanism of anorectal intercourse, usually results in denuding of the protecting cellular and mucous layer of rectum and anus. The physical act of intercourse leads to abrasions of the mucus lining and delivers pathogens directly to the crypts and columnar cells allowing easy entry.

2.3. HIV is known to deplete cell-mediated immunity by depletion of T cells and distraction of Langerhans cells. This allows, through unknown mechanisms, propagation of oncogenic process such as Human Papilloma Virus (HPV) to become dysplasia.

3. CLASSIFICATION SYSTEM FOR HIV AND AIDS

3.1. CD4 positive lymphocyte category
Category 1. Cells more than 500 cells.

Category 2. Cells between 200 to 400 cells.

Category 3. Cells less than 200 cells.

3.2. Clinical category A B C
Category A. HIV Positive, asymptomatic, persistent generalized lymph adenopathy.

Category B. Symptomatic conditions that are attributable to HIV or conditions that have clinical course or require management that is complicated by HIV infection.

Category C. Diagnosis included in AIDS surveillance case definition.

3.3. Nature of the disease
i. HIV immuno- suppression driven disease (casual).

ii. HIV associated diseases (linked without direct cause or effect).

iii. Independent disease (coincidental).

4. ANORECTAL LESIONS

The anorectal lesions in HIV patients are discussed under the following headings.

i. Perianal suppuration.

ii. Fissure.

iii. Haemorrhoids.

iv. Herpes Simplex (HSV).

v. Condyloma.

vi. Anal neoplasia.

vii. Kaposi's Sarcoma.

4.1. Perianal suppurations

The classical site of perianal suppuration is crypt infection occurring at dentate line. Spread occurring in a variable manner through the intersphinteric or trans sphincteric space and manifesting as a perianal abscess. Wide varieties of bacterial pathogens are reported in anorectal suppurations including Mycobacterium tuberculosis, mycobacterium avian. Because of lack of inflammatory cells in HIV patients, these infection are insidious may lack of the tell-tale erythema. Anal or rectal pain and fever are the presenting symptoms of perirectal suppuration and these abscess can be detected by rectal examination. Severe perianal sepsis causing marked tissue destruction may be one of the initial presenting features of AIDS. Recurrent sepsis and failure to respond to conventional therapy is common in AIDS. Metastatic sepsis and severe necrotizing gangrene is a well-known complication particularly in AIDS patients with low CD4 count.

Prompt drainage of the perianal or perirectal abscess must be done as earliest as possible to avoid further spread of the infection and other, complications thereafter. Conventional perianal drainage wound may heal within 8 weeks in 91% in AIDS patients.

4.2. Fissure

HIV positive patients develop fissure without any particular aetiology and so they are called "Idiopathic Ulcers"

4.2.1. These ulcers are characteristically associated with hypotonic sphincter and are located more proximal than the normal position of fissure. They are extremely aggressive, erode through the sphincter, and Trans sphincteric planes into the perirectal space.

Significant pain may present when pocketing of pus or faecal materials in the cavities caused by the erosive process. The patient may present with purulent discharge and bleeding. It may be in eccentric position than the normal position and may be multiples.

HIV associated anal ulcers can reliably differentiated from anal fissures and other ulcerations by a set of characteristic features described by VIAMONTE et al. These include noting the lesions, Sphincter tone, Sphincter or Post anal space involvement, Associated skin tag and Mucous bridging and the width of the ulcer base.

DIFFERENTIATING FEATURES (Viamonte etal)

S.no	Description	Benign anal ulcers	Idiopathic anal ulcers
1	Location	Low	High
2	Sphincter	Hypertonic	Lax
3	Sphincter invasion	No	Present
4	Sentinel skin tag	Present	No
5	Mucosal bridging	No	Present
6	Width	Narrow base	Broad base
7	AIDS	+/-50%	+100%

It is certainly possible for HIV patients to develop a typical anal fissure unrelated to their HIV disease.

4.2.2. Fissure or ulcer in HIV patients may be due to Syphilis, Tuberculosis, Herpes simplex, Cytomegalovirus, or Squamous cell carcinoma. In these cases the treatment must be directed to the underlying disease process rather than a simple local surgical therapy.

4.2.3. Surgical treatment

The surgical treatment of anal fissure in HIV patients, is modified by the following factors. i. intractable diarrhoea. ii. Degree of existing faecal incontinence. iii. The effect of the proposed surgical procedure on continence. Several surgeons have reported relief of HIV anal ulceration associated symptoms after surgical excision, despite poor healing and persistent wounds. Poor wound healing is associated with low CD4 cell count. HIV positive patients who have an atypical fissure or ulcer, in the absence of any other identifiable aetiology should be treated under anaesthesia with local debridement of the area and un roofing any pocket.

Continuous symptoms can be treated with intralesional injection of Depomedrol biweekly. Oral steroids prove almost as effective as intra lesion injection. In patients with hypertonic sphincter with sphincter spasm, in HIV positive, may be treated lateral internal sphincterotomy.

4.3. Haemorrhoids

Elective surgery for prolapsing haemorrhoids should be avoided except extremely healthy HIV positive patients, because healing may be prolonged. Asymptomatic HIV positive patients who not meet the clinical or CD4 count diagnostic criteria for AIDS can be treated with haemorrhoidectomy. AIDS patients with more advanced disease are at increased risk for wound healing problems. The benefits of symptomatic relief may still warranted the surgical treatment in these groups of patients.

4.4. Viral infection

Herpes Simplex virus (HSV) 1and 2. HSV infection occurs in Anorectal region in essentially passive homosexual men. The ulcerated lesions can be seen perianal, anal canal and rectum in patients with AIDS. Both biopsy and tissue culture yield a high positive rate. Anti-viral treatment is advised for one year.

4.5. Condyloma (anal warts)

Ano genital warts are the common sexually transmitted disease. Even in pre HIV era increased rates were described in male with homosexual. More recent investigation report that 3 to 24.9% of HIV positive patients have anal warts. The infective agent of anal condyloma is Human Papilloma Virus (HPV) a DNA Papova virus. Ulceration and dysplasia are common in condyloma. There is increased risk of dysplasia with HIV positive patients and condyloma localised above the dentate line. The incident of anal squamous cell carcinoma is more in homosexual men with AIDS is as high as 84 times that of general population. It reported that 12.2% of those with squamous cell carcinoma had concurrent

Condyloma and that 3.5% of those with condyloma had invasive carcinoma.

The clinical presentations of anal warts are variable, bleeding, itching, anal discomfort or present with perianal mass. Pain may not be the presenting symptom. Rectal examination and proctoscopic examination should be done because up to 78% will have internal lesions.

It is difficult to eradicate warts in HIV positive patients and the lesion may be extensive. Dysplasia is associated with HIV positive and diminished CD4 cell count. The amount of dysplasia is predictive of immune status but not the recurrence rate.

4.5.1. Podophyllin
Podophyllin with Tincture Benzoin 10 or 20% solution is applied with cotton wool swabs. After 5 to 10 minutes, it is washed with normal saline. It is repeated weekly for up to 3 months. It is produces irritation of the skin, local and systemic toxicity. Purified podophyllin toxin (Podofitox) has higher therapeutic effects than podophyllin itself.

4.5.2. Bichloroacetic acid and Trichloroacetic acid
When applied locally causes chemical burns destroying the keratin layers and expose tissue underneath. It requires neutralization with sodium bicarbonate. Multiple applications are required over a short period.

4.5.3. Chemotherapeutic agents
i. 5 fluorouracil (5FU) 5% cream for 7 days. 5FU with salicylic acid preparation called Soleoderm is now on use.

ii. Bleomycin is both antibiotics and anti tumourus agent.

4.5.4. Cryotherapy
Liquid Nitrogen is used through a special applicator.

4.5.5. Interferon
Its anti-proliferative property towards virus is effective in Condyloma. It is given intra lesion injection 3 times a week for 3 weeks.

4.5.6. SURGICAL TREATMENT

Wide excision, in the form of shaving the lesion with scalpel, Electro coagulation, Laser application, and excision by scissors. The excised specimen must be sent for Histopathological examination to exclude carcinoma in situ. It is advised aggressive treatment for anal condyloma in patients with early HIV positive or AIDS patients to reduce the morbidity caused by aggressive anal squamous cell carcinoma.

In HIV and AIDS patients, surgery should not be denied, when required because of risks of occupational transmission of HIV or AIDS and the fear of higher complication rate. Relief of symptoms, improvement in quality of life should be the chief consideration when treating these patients.

4.6. Anal neoplasm

Anal neoplasm is more prevalent in patients with AIDS and may present as fissure or fistulous abscess, emphasizing the need for aggressive biopsy from any suspicious lesions.

4.6.1. Anal intra epithelial neoplasia (AIN)

In Human Papilloma Virus (HPV) infection, HIV may be cofactor to induce anorectal dysplasia. Anal dysplasia and carcinoma in situ (CIS) are considered precursor to the development of invasive squamous cell carcinoma of the anus. These lesions are collectively referred as Anal Intracellular Neoplasia (AIN)

4.6.2. Condyloma accumulata

It is frequently found among HIV positive and (AIDS) patients. The malignancy transformation through AIN is 15%, which may progress to carcinoma in- situ and invasive anogenital squamous cell carcinoma often at an earlier age. Once AIN develops in HIV positive or AIDS patients the disease may advance more rapidly.

4.7 KAPOSI'S SARCOMA:

About 40 to 50 % of patients with AIDS develops these unusual sarcoma and it is the most common malignant tumour in patients with AIDS. This endothelial tumour has shown wide spread involvement of the skin, mucosa, lymph nodes and visceral organs. In both homosexual and bisexual men with AIDS, 43% have Kaposi's sarcoma.

CHAPTER 16

ANAL INTRAEPITHELIAL NEOPLASIA (AIN)

AIN is defined as presence of cellular and nuclear Abnormalities, in the anal canal and perianal epithelium, without a breach of the epithelial basement membrane. This condition is a precursor to some squamous cell carcinoma of the anus.

1. NOMENCLATURE OF AIN

1.1. The dysplastic lesions in the anal canal region were initially reported as mild, moderate, and severe by the pathologist.

However, as the connections between the anal dysplasia and Human Papilloma virus (HPV) was established, new criteria borrowing from cervical pathology classification system were developed, using the Bethesda system terminology AIN I, AIN II, and AIN III. This system led to uncertainty regarding the significance of AIN II lesions.

So a simpler system consisting of a two- tried approach of Low grade and High grade Squamous Intraepithelial lesions (LSIL and HSIL). Under this system AIN I corresponds to LSIL and AIN II, AIN III to HSIL. HSIL are considered pre malignant, whereas LSIL are not felt to be pre malignant, but DO have the potential to progress to HSIL. Cytology reports will occasionally include the term Atypical Squamous Cell of Undetermined Significance (ASCUS) that can be generally the LSIL category.

1.2. Unification of terms related to anal intra epithelial neoplasia.

LSIL. Condyloma or ASCUS, AIN I, Mild dysplasia.

HSIL. AIN II, Moderate dysplasia, AIN III Severe dysplasia.

2. RISK FACTORS

2.1. High risk sexual behaviour
Most commonly occurs in men who has sex with men (MSM), receptive anal intercourse, or multiple sexual partners have been shown to be associated with high rate of HSIL.

2.2. HIV infection
The clue that the HIV population was at particular risk for AIN came with the findings that anal canal carcinoma rates have notably increased in HIV era, compared to pre HIV era. Infection with HIV is associated with an increased risk of AIN in all infected persons and particularly in MSM populations and thus elevated risk for AIN in the HIV positive populations has been demonstrated in surgical studies. The reason for the increased risk for AIN in HIV positive persons is likely because both are associated with Human Papilloma Virus (HPV), inability to clean HPV infection and for simultaneous infections with multiple strains of HPV.

2.3. Human Papilloma Virus (HPV)
The HPV family includes double-striated DNA viruses that infect mucosal and cutaneous epithelium and induce cellular proliferation. HPV has been shown to be casually associated with anogenital neoplasia, including AIN and anal cancer. The histological transitional zone, as in cervix, is the most common site of the Histopathological changes associated with HPV infection.

2.4. Other risk factors
2.4.1. When considering an individual's risk for AIN and anal squamous cell carcinoma (SCC), a personal history of cervical intra epithelial

neoplasia (CIN), and gynaecological cancer should be elucidated by the clinician, since a history of genital neoplasia is a risk factor for anal neoplasm.

2.4.2. The presence of HPV related dysplasia in other anatomical regions in an individual is a well-established risk factor for AIN. Since the development of HPV related malignancy implies chronic infection with an oncogenic HPV strain thus increasing the risk.

2.4.3. Immuno suppression
Chronic immuno suppression is a risk factor for the development of AIN and for the progression of AIN to cancer.

3. AIN FOLLOWS UP STUDY

AIN is assumed to be the precursor lesions of the anal cancer. Some cases of LSIL progress to HSIL and then to SCC. AIN is common in high-risk population. Spontaneous regression from HSIL to LSIL and LSIL to normal has been reported in some cases.

4. CLINICAL PRESENTATION

AIN is neither visible nor palpable and frequently symptomless. The patient may present with anal or perianal condyloma, pruritus and bleeding. Most patients with perianal lesions have involvement of anal transitional zone.

5. Diagnosis

5.1. Anal cytology
Anal cytology is used in screening for AIN. The technique of anal cytology consists of inserting a water moistened polyester fibre swabs into the rectum and removing the swabs in a twisting manner allow the sampling of the transitional zone and anal canal. The swab is processed using a liquid cytology technique prior to the Papanicolaou staining

and then the pathologist study the smear. Sampling can be done by the patients themselves or by the attending surgeon.

5.2. High Resolution Anoscope (HRA)

If abnormal cytology is detected with anal cytological study, the next step is to localize the source of atypical cells by HRA.

The HRA consists of examining the squamo columnar junction, anal canal and perianal skin under magnification using a colposcope (and acetic acid staining) The anoscope is placed into the anus with lignocaine lubricants, a swab soaked in 3 to 5% acetic acid solution is inserted into the anal canal, the anoscope is removed and the swab is kept sometimes in the anus and then removed. Acetic acid application causes an "Acetowhite" change in area of abnormal transitional epithelium. The mucosa is carefully examined for any mucosal abnormalities including flat or slightly raised area of thickened mucosa with or without vascular pattern abnormalities. Lugol's iodine is applied in similar way, but in this case, the concerning lesions failed to stain with iodine (Lugol's negative) because iodine is glycophilic and dysplastic tissues lack glycogen and appear thick mustard colour. Any suspicious lesions, including condyloma, atypical surface configuration, mosaicism or atypical blood vessels are biopsied under direct visualization. Area with colour changes seen on acetic acid staining and are subsequently found to be Lugols negative are highly suspicious of dysplasia. HRA is considered superior to standard anoscope. In addition to detection of AIN, HRA also facilitates the application of treatment targeting AIN. HRA is ideally performed at centres specializing in its use rather than at clinics lacking trained experts.

5.3. NOVAL IMAGING

Technology may identify high-risk lesions without the need for tissue biopsy. Confocal laser microscopy, which has been shown as effective as for detection of superficial oesophageal squamous cell carcinoma, might be useful for the detection and grading of AIN.

6. MANAGEMENT OF AIN

Because AIN can be misdiagnosed and can be progressed to carcinoma in some, yet regress in others, expert centres are best equipped to determine which individual should be treated and what treatment modalities should be considered. The management strategies are dependent upon the extent of the lesion. AIN I and AIN II are unlikely to progress, so conservative approach of regular review for about 2 years. If the lesion remains unchanged both clinically and by biopsy and the patient is not immuno compromised, the patient may be discharged from outpatient care. However, regular review should be continued at 6 months interval in immuno-compromised patients. Patient must be advised to come when any change in the lesion or symptoms. or occurrence.

Highly Active Anti-Retroviral Therapy (HAART) has proven effective for HIV patients but it has little effect on the anal cytological appearance in AIN.

6.1. Topical therapy

Topical therapy consists of direct application of medications to specific lesion.

Trichloroacetic acid (TCA), 5- Fluorouracil (5 FU) and the Immune modulator Imiquimod are used in topical therapy. TCA is well tolerated, can be applied without specialized equipment and is effective. AlN Lesion of HSIL regresses to LSIL or complete resolution in 71to79% of cases. Treatment with 5FU reported 39% of complete clearance, 17% partial response, and 37% no response. 50% of the complete responders had recurrence of AIN at 6 months. Imiquimod therapy with (5%cream) had 61% sustained response at 36 months. Topical therapy appears to be well tolerated and has reasonably effective. Topical therapy may be best utilized as an adjunct to local ablative therapy.

6.2. Local ablative therapy

6.2.1. Local ablative therapy consists of targeted destruction therapy. Most commonly used techniques are Radio Frequency Ablation (RFA) or electro cautery. Both RFA and electro cautery therapy are associated with minimal morbidity, particularly with a greater number of treatment sessions. RFA is applied to the anal mucosa to treat AlN is safe and tolerable. But evidence of treatment efficacy is limited.

6.2.2. Electro cautery therapy

Electro cautery therapy has been studied more extensively. Increased success was seen in those patients with 2 to 4 sessions compared to those treated with only one session.

6.3. HPV Vaccine

Infection with HPV is now reorganized to be responsible for nearly all cervical cancers, and 95% of anal cancer. There are 100 types of HPV that infect humans, and about 50% infection in ano genital tract. Some of the subtypes are commonly found in anogenital cancers and they are called "High risk", "Intermediate" group and "Low risk" strains of HPV. HPV type 16 and 18 and to a lesser extent 6 and 11, are primarily oncogenic strains found in anal cancer. The discovery of these strains led to certain vaccines targeting them. The first vaccine was against HPV types 16 and 18, followed by the quadrivalent vaccine targeting types 6, 11, and 16 and 18. A recent study shows 75 % reduction in LSIL and HSIL. Vaccination is also appears to be effective in preventing recurrent in high AIN. Further studies provide strong evidence that HPV vaccination is effective in preventing progress of AIN and cancer.

7. SURGICAL TREATMENT

Surgery for AIN is associated with significant morbidity, often requiring large area of excision of the healthy tissue and yet is associated with a high recurrence rate. As recurrence of AIN is presumably mediated by on-going exposure to predisposing risk factors, notably on-going HPV infection. Further, the improvement in local therapy outcome, surgical treatment for AIN is not recommended as a routine treatment option.

7.1. Indications for surgery

Operative treatment is indicated when there is a visible or palpable lesion in the anus or perianal region (AIN III). There is risk of developing frank carcinoma. In immuno compromised individuals there may be a delay is wound healing after surgery.

7.2. Biopsy of the lesion to confirm the diagnosis is mandatory. Four quadrant punch Biopsy (using 4 mm corneal punch) around the anus and in the anal canal to determine the extent of the AIN III (mapping procedure). Histologically the lesion maybe more extensive than the clinical appearance of the lesion. In AIN III lesions that occupy more than 50% of the anal circumference, needs local excision with or without rotation flap to close the defect depending upon the area of defect. For more extensive lesion CO_2 Laser vaporization or Cryosurgery may proceeds the surgical excision may be grafting. In spite of grossly apparent complete excision there is risk of incomplete excision oncologically, and recurrence may occur.

7.3. Outcome of surgery

Surgical treatment may lead to extensive surgery with significant morbidity including painful recovery, wound care, and anal stenosis. In AIN III lesions recurrence occurs in 80 % of cases within 12 months. Follow up anal Papanicolaou screening has 65-90% sensitivity and30-60percentage specificity for the diagnosis of AIN. Anal intraepithelial neoplasia is the precursor lesions to squamous cell cancer of the anus. The actual risk of progression remains unclear. But it has been shown, that the progression risk is elevated in certain high risk groups including

i. Those with persistent infection with high-risk HPV strains.

ii. HIV positive individual with low CD4 counts.

iii. MSM.

iv. Individual with the history of HPV mediated genetic cancers particularly cervical cancer.

AIN can be challenging for diagnosis and treatment, it is better to refer to an expert centre where all specialists are available for proper management.

CHAPTER 17

CARCINOMA OF ANAL REGION

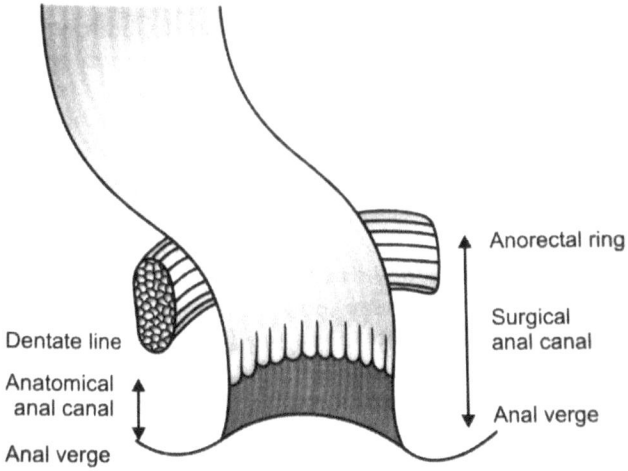

17.01. Anal canal (Anatomical and Surgical.)

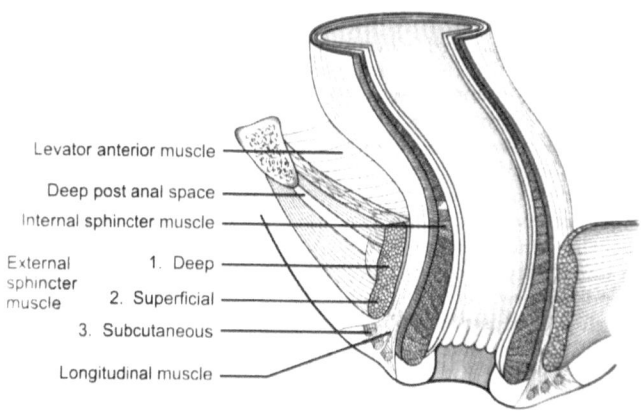

17.02. Anatomy of anal sphincters

Carcinoma of the anus differs from carcinoma of the rectum in histological structure, behaviour, and type of treatment. This is mainly because of its accessibility, abundant lymphatic drainage both superficial and deep, and its sensitivity to radiation. Most of the anal neoplasms are delayed in diagnosis, due to confusion with more common benign conditions. The common type of cancer in anal region is squamous cell carcinoma. It accounts for 2-3% of all tumours of the distal alimentary tract. Most of the anal cancer is curable by either primary chemo- radiation or local excision allowing sphincter preservation.

1. ANATOMICAL CONSIDERATION

1.1. The anal canal is 2.5 to 3 cm length and the Perianal region measures 6 cm from the anal verge (fig20.01). The anatomical landmarks for examination of this region are i. Anorectal ring, ii. The dentate line iii. The anal verge.

1.2. According to the traditional definition, the surgical anal canal extends from the anorectal ring (upper portion of the Puborectalis/ levator ani complex) at the floor of the pelvis to the anal verge (fig20.02). WHO have defined the anal canal as extending from anal verge to the lower border of the internal sphincter, which approximates with the above clinical definition.

1.3. The lymphatic drainage in this region unfortunately, is diffuse from the dentate line and within the anal canal; the spread of cancer in this region may be in three directions, upwards to the superior haemorrhoidal system, laterally along the middle haemorrhoidal system, and down ward to the inguinal nodes.

1.4. The lining of the anal canal is divided into three zones.

i. Colorectal zone.

ii. Anal transitional zone.

iii. Squamous zone.

In colorectal zone, the lining layer consists of columnar mucosal type identical to distal rectal mucosa. The Anal Transitional Zone (ATZ) extending approximately, one cm upwards from the dentate line. The ATZ contains many epithelial variants, including colorectal mucosa, squamous cell as well as the ATZ epithelium made up of 4to 9 cell layers including Basal, Columnar, and Cuboid cells. Melanocytes and endocrine cells are also occasionally found. The squamous zone extending from dentate line to anal verge and consists of unkeratinizing squamous mucosa without skin appendages. Melanocytes may be present in this squamous zone.

1.5. The anal verge is the point at which modified squamous cell epithelium (anoderm) of the anal canal meets hair bearing perianal skin. The anal margin refers to the perianal skin extending approximately 5to6 cm from the anal verge. The Perianal skin contains Sweat, Sebaceous, and Apocrine glands, and is keratinized. Essentially all skin cancer can affect the anal margin.

1.6. Lymphatic drainage

a. The lymphatic drainage from colorectal zone and ATZ is primarily upwards to the inferior mesenteric nodes via superior rectal lymphatic. To a lesser degree, drainage may occur via the inferior and middle rectal lymphatic to the internal iliac nodes.

b. The lymphatic drainage of the anal canal between the dentate line and anal verge (squamous zone) is predominately to the inguinal lymph nodes. Secondary drainage occurs via inferior rectal lymphatic to the ischiorectal nodes and internal iliac nodes.

c. The lymphatic drainage from anal margin and perianal skin is entirely to the inguinal nodes.

2. PRE MALIGNANT LESIONS AND PREDISPOSING FACTORS

2.1. Anal Intraepithelial Neoplasia (AIN) is a precancerous lesion. Histologically it is classified as AIN I, AIN II, and AIN III. The AIN

III has the histological appearance of cancer in situ. AIN is found in association with HIV infection.

2.2. HIV
The HIV epidemic and prolonged survival due to Highly Active Anti-Retroviral therapy (HAART) have resulted in a dramatic increase in the incidence of anal cancer among HIV positive patients, predominately in men who have sex with men(MSM), and at younger age.

2.3. Genital Warts
Genital warts due to Human Papilloma Virus (HPV) transmission of HPV occurs through repetitive anal sex.

2.4. Bowens disease
There is evidence that perianal Bowen's disease is similar to anal cancer insitu (CIS) and is well established that the Bowen's disease is pre malignant lesion. The histological appearance is characteristic with atypical epithelial cells involving the full thickness of epidermis. In addition, the cells with large halo hyper chromic nuclei the so-called Bowenoid cells are often seen.

2.5. Paget's disease
Perianal Paget's disease may be either Primary (insitu or with an invasive component) or secondary essentially downward Pagetoid extension from an established adenocarcinoma. Clinically perianal Paget's presents as slowly enlarging eczematous, erythematous, scaly rash, which is often sharply demarcated.

2.6. Long standing perianal fistula may predispose for malignancy

2.7. Other predisposing factors
Lympho Granuloma Venerium (LGV), Herpes simplex virus type 2, Condylomata and Chlamydia.

3. CARCINOMA OF ANAL MARGIN AND PERIANAL MARGIN

(Squamous zone of anal canal).

3.1. Carcinoma of the anal margin is 4 times more common in men than women. These tumours are distal to the dentate line, the transition of hairless anal canal to the hair containing perianal skin but less than 5cm from anal verge and they are Squamous cell carcinoma. In perianal carcinoma, the cancer is arising from the perianal skin more than 5 cm from the anal verge.

3.2. Variants of squamous cell carcinoma include Cloacogenic, Transitional, and Basaloid tumours are collectively known as epidermoid carcinoma. According to WHO classification these variants are now referred to as

i.   Large cell keratinizing,

ii. Large cell non keratinizing (transitional) and

iii. Basaloid.

These tumours directly involve the adjacent anal sphincters in 50% of the patients and inguinal node involvement in 1/3rd of cases. Histologically, mostly of keratinising variety with nests of keratin in the masses of squamous cells known as" Epithelial Pearl". Bowen's disease, Paget's disease, and Basal carcinoma, are also occur in this zone. Carcinoma of anal margin has a better prognosis than that of anal canal.

4. SQUAMOUS CELL CARCINOMA OF THE ANAL CANAL

Anal canal cancer is occurs more in female (3: 2) the tumour arises from the area between the dentate line and normal rectal mucosa above. The tumours are mostly small but ulcerating confined to one segment of the anal canal, rarely forming semi annular or annular. The tumour may involve sphincter muscles and involves the vagina in female resulting in fistula.

4.1. Histologically, anal canal malignancy may be classified as

i. Epidermoid squamous cell.

ii. Muco epidermoid.

iii. Transitional - Cloacogenic carcinoma (Basaloid).

iv. Adenocarcinoma.

v. Malignant melanoma.

5. TRANSITIONAL

Cloacogenic carcinoma. It resembles carcinoma of the urothelium to certain extent or it may have a pattern to that of Basal cell carcinoma of the skin and hence the term Basaloid because the cells at periphery are arranged in an orderly palisade fashion. These tumours may appear as a low-grade malignancy and have a better prognosis; however, they are metastasizing tumours. They do not behave as the common Basal cell carcinoma of the skin.

6. SYMPTOMS

The symptoms of anal canal carcinoma include

i. Rectal bleeding.

ii. Mucus discharge.

iii. Pruritus.

iv. Sensation of a lump in the anus.

v. Tenesmus.

vi. Disturbances in continence.

vii. Change in bowel habits.

Tenesmus implies invasion of the anal sphincter. Delay in diagnosis is common in many cases as the symptoms are confused with those of common benign conditions. The disease may be obscured by the presence of fistula or painful fissure. Occasionally histological examination of excised haemorrhoids may reveal the malignancy.

7. CLINICAL EXAMINATION

Rectal examination will reveal the lesion and its physical character. The lesion may extend up wards involving the rectum. In other way a down ward spread of rectal cancer, can present as anal cancer (17.1). Some lesions may fungate through the anal canal and present as fistula with atypical findings.

8. EVALUATION

i. Rectal examination- to find out, the exact local and perianal indurations.
ii. Proctoscopy- to see the lesion and to take Biopsy for confirmation of cancer
iii. Colonoscopy- to rule out proximal lesions.
iv. CT - for the evaluation of lymph node involvement.
v. MRI, PET SCAN(Positron Emission Tomography) -for the study of depth of tumour invasion.
vi. Blood tests particularly for HIV and AIDS.

A combination of AIDS and anal cancer is often an Over whelming problem for the patient and for the surgeon.

9. ASSESSMENT OF PROGNOSIS

i. Longer the duration of symptoms poorer the prognosis.
ii. Epidermoid carcinoma of anal region is asymptomatic and has a favourable prognosis.

iii. Prognosis of epidermoid carcinoma is directly related to the size of the primary tumour.
iv. Tumour at anal margin has better prognosis than those of anal canal.
v. Keratinizing tumour has a little better prognosis.
vi. Carcinoma in a fistula tract has poor prognosis.

Although the squamous cell carcinoma of the anus is often said to be a loco regional disease, distant metastasis does occur, primarily to the liver. It is reported 40% of patients whose initial treatment with chemo radiation failed, died with metastatic disease.

10. STAGING

10.1. Staging - Modified ABC classification.
Stage A. Invasion of mucosa and sub mucosa.

Stage B. Sphincter muscle involvement.

    B1. Invasion of internal sphincter.

    B2. Invasion of external sphincter.

    B3. Invasion beyond sphincter, into the adjacent tissues.

Stage C. Lymph node involvement.

This modification of ABC classification has prognostic (17.2) significance of both survival and incidence of local recurrence.

10.2. Ultra-sonogram classification. Endo anal ultra-sonogram can accurately determine the depth of penetration of the lesion preoperatively.

i. uT1. Tumour confined to the sub mucosa.
ii. uT2 a. Tumour invaded the internal sphincter.
iii. uT2 b. Tumour invaded the external sphincter.
iv. uT3. Tumour invaded through both sphincters into the perianal tissue.
v. uT4. Tumour invaded the adjacent structures.

11. TREATMENT OF ANAL CANCER

A combined modality treatment is the first line of treatment for anal cancer. The combined modality therapy, although originally intended as neo adjuvant therapy prior to Abdomino Perianal Resection(APR), the unexpected finding of a complete pathological response in majority of patients led to the use of APR only for patients with biopsy proven residual disease at the completion of therapy. This results in historical paradigm shift after mid 1970 from mutilating primary radical surgery (APR) with colostomy, to a highly effective and sphincter saving chemo-radiation(NIGRO). Radical surgery is reserved as a salvage approach for this treatment failure. Now the management of anal cancer should be considered as a team effort by the surgeons, radiotherapists and medical oncologists to define the most appropriate treatment strategies for each case.

Earlier 1985 the conventional therapy for anal squamous cell carcinoma was abdomino Perianal resection, and local excision reserved for small early tumours. Recently the combination of chemotherapy and radiotherapy has become the standard treatment. In planning the surgical treatment, the most important consideration is whether the growth extends up to involve the rectal mucosa proper or confined to the anal canal and perianal skin. Surgery may consist of strictly local excision of growth bearing rectum and greater part of anal canal or may include rectal excision by perineum or APR depending upon the site and extent of the lesion.

11.1. Indications for surgery
i.   Chemotherapy intolerances.
ii. Residual tumour after completion of Nigro protocol.
iii. Adenocarcinoma after neo adjuvant chemo radiation.
iv. Recurrent tumour after initial complete response to Nigro protocol.
v.   Chemo radiation treatment refractory but symptomatic lesions.
vi. Diversion colostomy in persistent disease or treatment sequelae.

vii. Perianal and anal canal margin squamous cell carcinoma as per skin cancer treatment.

viii. Watch full waiting, possible Re excision for incidental cancer in Condyloma excision or haemorrhoidectomy specimen, intraepithelial carcinoma (cancer insitu), verucous carcinoma. Surgery for residual disease after chemo radiation appears better prognosis than after locally recurrent disease.

12. COMBINED MODALITY THERAPY (CHEMO RADIATION THERAPY)

12.1. Nigro Protocol. For T2 and T 3 anal cancer

i. 5 FU-750 mg/ m2 infusion on days 1to 4 and during the last week of radiation therapy.

ii. Mitomycin C 15 mg/ m2 IV on day I.

iii. 45-59 Gy in daily dose of 200 CGy for 5 days a week for five weeks. Radiation evaluated after 45 Gy. If necessary, dose may be increased further radiation up to 59 Gy.

12.2. In some centres Mitomycin C is replaced by Cisplatinum with a dose of 80-100 mg/ m2 on day one. Some other centres have used Bleomycin or Adriamycin.

Norwegian Radium hospital OSLO, draw a conclusion that the treatment regime is effective but carries a significant risk of complications.

12.3. Complications of Nigro protocol

a. Acute toxicity
  i. Mylo suppression.
  ii. Cardio pulmonary toxicity
  iii. Anoproctitis.
  iv. Perianal dermatitis.
  v. Diarrhoea.

B. Late complications.

    i. Anorectal ulceration.

    ii. Leucopoenia.

    iii. Thrombocytopenia.

    iv. Anal incontinence.

    v. Anal stenosis.

    vi. Chronic pelvic pain.

    vii. Alopecia.

13. PHOTO DYNAMIC THERAPY (PDT)

PDT is a technique with a potential for localization by Fluorescence and selective destruction of malignant tumour, particularly small multifocal lesions. It is based on the systemic administration of certain sensitizing drugs which are retained with some selectivity by tumours which can be activated by laser or non-laser light to produce a local cytotoxic effect.

14. TREATMENT OF INGUINAL LYMPH NODES

Groin nodes involvement may be up to 40%. Inguinal metastasis is slightly higher with anal margin than with anal canal lesions. The treatment of inguinal block dissection is probably preferable as it is for the cervical lymph node secondary in cases of cancer lip or tongue. Radiotherapy is reserved for cases with fixed inoperable nodes. Removal of single node or 2 or 3 for diagnostic purposes not likely to be helpful. If the clinical suspicion on metastasis arose, do formal block dissection.

When the nodes are involved by secondary, they should be removed to prevent ulceration, pain due to malignant infiltration of the femoral nerve and bleeding due to infiltration of femoral vessels.

15. ANORECTAL MELANOMA

Anorectal melanoma occurs less than 1% of all colorectal malignancies. Melanoma in colorectal region is the third most common site, after skin and ocular. Physical examination may reveal a pigmented, polypoidal lesion. It may appear as a benign polyp or thrombosed haemorrhoids.

About 30 to, 70% of anorectal melanomas are amelanotic making clinical and histological diagnosis more difficult.

The treatment of anorectal melanoma is primarily surgical, as these lesions do not respond to radiation or chemotherapy. Wide local excision as an initial treatment is probably reasonable if local control can be obtained. Abdomino Perianal resection is reserved for cases in which local control is not possible with wide local excision.

16. ANAL ADENOCARCINOMA

WHO classified adenocarcinoma of anal region into three types based on presumed origin.

i. Rectal types.

ii. Anal gland and duct tape.

iii. Arising from chronic anorectal fistula.

Tumours arising from the colorectal mucosa lining of the proximal anal canal behaves as distal rectal cancer and treated accordingly.

The anal glands are lined by mucin secreting, stratified columnar epithelium and open into the anal canal via the ducts at the level of the dentate line. Tumours originating from the anal glands are often located in the ischiorectal space without involvement of the underlying anal mucosa.

Anal adenocarcinoma from chronic anorectal fistula, the presenting symptoms are nonspecific and are similar to common benign anal conditions and accurate diagnosis is often delayed.

16.1. The treatment of adenocarcinoma in anal region is depending upon the size and extent of the lesion, wide local excision or abdomino Perianal resection is adopted. The role of radiation and chemotherapy as the primary treatment has yet to be defined. The role of adjuvant chemo radiation is also not clear.

A common theme in most anal neoplasm appears, due to confusion with more common benign condition. The clinician must maintain a high index of suspicion when evaluating lesions of the anal canal and anal margin.

www.ingramcontent.com/pod-product-compliance
Lightning Source LLC
Chambersburg PA
CBHW020903180526
45163CB00007B/2605